ABC OF MAJOR TRAUMA

ABC OF MAJOR TRAUMA

Second Edition

edited by

DAVID SKINNER FRCS
Consultant in accident and emergency medicine, Oxford Radcliffe Hospital

PETER DRISCOLL FRCS
Consultant in accident and emergency medicine, Hope Hospital, Salford

and

RICHARD EARLAM FRCS
Consultant in general surgery, Royal London Hospital

BMJ
Publishing
Group

© BMJ Publishing Group 1991, 1996

All rights reserved. No part of this publication may be reproduced, stored in a retrieval system, or transmitted, in any form or by any means, electronic, mechanical, photocopying, recording and/or otherwise, without the prior written permission of the publishers.

First published in 1991
Second edition 1996
by the BMJ Publishing Group, BMA House, Tavistock Square, London WC1H 9JR

British Library Cataloguing in Publication Data

A catalogue record for this book is available from the British Library

ISBN 0-7279-0917-7

Typeset by Apek Typesetters Ltd., Nailsea, Bristol
Printed in Singapore by Craft Print

Contents

		Page
Foreword		vii
Preface to the first edition		viii
Preface to the second edition		ix
Acknowledgments for illustrations		x

1 Initial assessment and management—I: primary survey PETER DRISCOLL, *consultant in accident and emergency medicine, Hope Hospital, Salford, and* DAVID SKINNER, *consultant in accident and emergency medicine, Oxford Radcliffe Hospital*   **1**

2 Initial assessment and management—II: secondary survey PETER DRISCOLL *and* DAVID SKINNER   **6**

3 The upper airway DAVID WATSON, *consultant anaesthetist and senior lecturer in anaesthesia and intensive care medicine, Homerton and St Bartholomew's Hospitals, London*   **11**

4 Chest injuries STEPHEN ROONEY, *cardiac transplant fellow, Queen Elizabeth Medical Centre, Birmingham,* STEPHEN WESTABY, *consultant cardiothoracic surgeon, Oxford Radcliffe Hospital, and* TIMOTHY GRAHAM, *consultant cardiothoracic surgeon, Queen Elizabeth Medical Centre*   **15**

5 Hypovolaemic shock PETER J F BASKETT, *consultant anaesthetist, Royal Infirmary and Frenchay Hospital, Bristol*   **22**

6 Head injuries ROSS BULLOCK, *Lind Lawrence associate professor of neurological surgery, West Hospital, Richmond, Virginia, USA, and* GRAHAM TEASDALE, *professor of neurosurgery, University of Glasgow*   **28**

7 Maxillofacial injuries IAIN HUTCHISON, *consultant in maxillofacial surgery, Royal London Hospital,* MICHAEL LAWLOR, *consultant in maxillofacial surgery, Northbrook Clinic, Dublin, and* DAVID SKINNER   **36**

8 Spine and spinal cord ANDREW SWAIN, *consultant in accident and emergency medicine, General Hospital, Weston-super-Mare,* JOHN DOVE, *consultant, Stoke on Trent Spinal Service, and* HARRY BAKER, *consultant in rehabilitation medicine, Rookwood Hospital, Cardiff*   **41**

9 Abdomen ANDREW COPE, *consultant in accident and emergency medicine, Peterborough District Hospital, Cambridgeshire, and* WILLIAM STEBBINGS, *consultant in general surgery, St Mark's Hospital for Diseases of the Rectum and Colon, London*   **49**

10 The urinary tract TIMOTHY TERRY, *consultant urologist, Leicester General Hospital, and* ANTHONY DEANE, *consultant urologist, William Harvey Hospital, Ashford, Kent, and Buckland Hospital, Dover, Kent*   **54**

11 Limb injuries KEITH M WILLET, *consultant orthopaedic surgeon, Oxford Radcliffe Hospital,* RAYMOND ROSS, *consultant orthopaedic surgeon, Hope Hospital, Salford,* HUGH DORRELL, *consultant in orthopaedic surgery, Lister Hospital, Stevenage, and* PETER KELLY, *consultant in accident and emergency medicine, Lister Hospital, Stevenage*   **60**

12 **Medical problems**   T D WARDLE, *consultant physician, Countess of Chester Hospital, Chester, and* PETER DRISCOLL   66

13 **Radiological assessment**   N M PERRY, *consultant radiologist, St Bartholomew's Hospital, and* M D LEWARS, *consultant radiologist, Southend General Hospital, and* PETER DRISCOLL   71

14 **Role of the trauma nurse**   LISA HADFIELD-LAW, *SDU manager, accident and emergency department, Oxford Radcliffe Hospital, and* ANDREW KENT, *charge nurse, department of emergency medicine, Hope Hospital, Salford*   80

15 **Scoring systems**   D W YATES, *professor of accident and emergency medicine, Hope Hospital, Salford*   83

16 **Handling distressed relatives and breaking bad news**   C A J McLAUCHLAN, *consultant in accident and emergency medicine, Royal Devon and Exeter Hospital, Exeter*   88

17 **Trauma in pregnancy**   PAMELA NASH, *consultant in accident and emergency medicine, Hillingdon Hospital, Middlesex, and* PETER DRISCOLL   93

18 **Paediatric trauma**   A R LLOYD-THOMAS, *consultant paediatric anaesthetist, Hospital for Sick Children, Great Ormond Street, London, and* I ANDERSON, *consultant in accident and emergency medicine, Victoria Infirmary, Glasgow*   97

19 **Trauma in the elderly**   CARL L GWINNUTT, *consultant anaesthetist, Hope Hospital, Salford, and* MICHAEL A HORAN, *professor of geriatric medicine, University of South Manchester*   107

20 **Prehospital care**   CARL L GWINNUTT, ALASTAIR W WILSON, *clinical director of accident and emergency medicine, Royal London Hospital, and* PETER DRISCOLL   111

21 **Transportation to hospital**   CARL GWINNUTT, ALASTAIR W WILSON, *and* PETER DRISCOLL   115

22 **Management of severe burns**   COLIN ROBERTSON, *consultant in accident and emergency medicine, Royal Infirmary, Edinburgh, and* OLIVER FENTON, *consultant plastic surgeon, Pinderfield Hospital, Wakefield*   118

23 **Chemical incidents**   VIRGINIA MURRAY, *honorary consultant occupational toxicologist, National Poisons Unit, Guy's Hospital, London*   124

24 **Blast and gunshot injuries**   TIM HODGETTS, *consultant in emergency medicine, Frimley Park Hospital, Surrey,* IAN HAYWOOD, *formerly professor of military Surgery, Royal Army Medical College, London,* JIM RYAN, *visiting professor of trauma, University College Hospital, London, and* DAVID SKINNER   127

25 **Trauma in hostile environments**   C J CAHILL, *consultant in accident and emergency medicine, Royal Naval Hospital, Gosport, Hampshire, and* VANESSA LLOYD-DAVIES, *military primary care physician, Cambridge Military Hospital, Aldershot, Hampshire*   131

26 **Major incidents**   TIM HODGETTS, *and* STEPHEN MILES, *consultant in accident and emergency medicine, Royal Hospitals Trust, London*   135

Index   141

FOREWORD

In December 1990 I wrote a foreword to the first edition of this book. At that time the Royal College of Surgeons of England's report on the management of major injuries, published in 1988, was beginning to have an impact on the way the seriously injured were managed in the United Kingdom. By 1990 its five major recommendations were at various stages of implementation. Training programmes for paramedics were under development and a pilot trauma centre was being established and evaluated at Stoke on Trent and compared with comparator centres in Preston and Hull. The Advanced Trauma Life Support programme was already well established by the royal college at instructor and provider level and a national audit of the outcomes of serious injury, the Major Trauma Outcome Study, was funded by the Department of Health and subscribed to by an increasing number of hospitals. Many of those interested in the management of the seriously injured were meeting regularly under the auspices of the newly established British Trauma Society.

All these activities were evidence of an increased interest in the fate of the seriously injured, both in terms of the way they were managed and the outcomes that were achieved. At that time I hailed this book as a concise and readable reference book which would guide and stimulate those who were involved in the treatment of the injured, or who planned to make the management of trauma their lifetime career.

Five years later, where has all this activity got us? As one who has had a lifetime interest in trauma management, I am pleased to report that I believe there has been a radical change for the better. It is now generally accepted that concentration of the management of the seriously injured in the hands of those who are interested in the problem and who are willing to provide an immediate high quality service is in the best interests of the patient. Also it is now accepted that comparative audit can indicate variations in outcome and stimulate changes that will improve performance. ATLS training is now accepted and so valued that the royal college is considering making it mandatory for all those who wish to take their examinations. The British Trauma Society is thriving.

The past five years have also seen the increasing influence of another report that was issued in 1988. That year the House of Lords committee on science and technology, in its report on priorities in medical research, proposed among other things, the evaluation of clinical practice and the dissemination and implementation of research results within the NHS. The National Health Service research and development directorate, which resulted from this report, has stimulated a move towards evidence based clinical practice. Just as in 1990 we were in a period of change in the structure of trauma services, so now we are in the midst of a period of evaluation, not only of the treatments given, but the way services are provided. Evidence based medical practice research is assessing the process and outcome in areas of uncertainty such as the value of on site intravenous fluid administration to the seriously injured and the prevention of venous thromboembolism.

This updated edition of the *ABC of Major Trauma* will continue to act as a valuable reference for those called on to treat the seriously injured. At the same time it recognises areas of uncertainty which need further research so that future editions of this book will be based on sound evidence of clinical effectiveness.

Professor of Surgery
Hope Hospital
University of Manchester

PROFESSOR SIR MILES IRVING

PREFACE TO THE FIRST EDITION

The management of patients with major injuries in the United Kingdom has been the subject of much discussion and debate over the past five years. The report of the Royal College of Surgeons of England highlighted various areas where medical management was substantially suboptimal; patients who should have survived did not do so because of poor management. The report also emphasised that experienced consultants in various specialties must become more involved in emergency treatment.

The chapter on initial assessment gives a sequential method of management that can be followed by one doctor if he or she is unfortunate enough to be working in isolation. Recent evidence suggests that a "trauma team" approach provides more speedy diagnosis and resuscitation and decreases mortality and morbidity. The same tasks must be completed but they can be allocated to different members of the team in order that the initial assessment is more rapid.

In the instructions on management we and many of the contributors have been influenced by the advanced trauma life support (ATLS) course, as originated by the American College of Surgeons and, more recently, run in the United Kingdom under the auspices of the Royal College of Surgeons of England. We believe that such a system will save lives and therefore have promoted a similar approach.

The various other chapters deal with specific problems related to one part of the body or with particular sorts of injuries, such as burns and blast injuries, or situations where large numbers of casualties are involved. We thank the authors for their efforts in producing a book which will, we hope, be of help to all those treating patients with major trauma. We also thank Fiona Whimster for encouragement and secretarial help.

DAVID SKINNER
PETER DRISCOLL
RICHARD EARLAM

December 1990

PREFACE TO THE SECOND EDITION

The past five years have seen significant changes in how injuries to separate and multiple body systems are managed. Furthermore, training in trauma care is now considered an integral part of a doctor's preparation for a career in anaesthetics, emergency medicine, or surgery. There has also been development of trauma training courses for nurses as well as staff working in the prehospital environment. Indeed many hospitals in the UK have incorporated several of these changes and developed multi-specialty trauma teams to optimise the care of the injured patient.

This second edition therefore provides a pertinent update on all the topics covered previously. Our aim, however, is to go further. With this edition we have taken the opportunity of incorporating several completely new aspects of trauma care. These include the management of medical problems in trauma patients, inter-hospital transfers, and trauma care in elderly people and hostile environments. The important role of the trauma nurse also forms an entirely new chapter.

We have endeavoured to ensure that this second edition remains relevant to all health care professionals involved in the chain of trauma care. If we have succeeded then it is in no small part due to the many people who have provided us with helpful advice over the past 5 years. Above all we are indebted to the authors of the individual chapters as well as to the continued support of the BMJ Publishing Group, and particularly to Deborah Reece. Without all their hard work and dedication this book could not have been written.

DAVID SKINNER
PETER DRISCOLL
RICHARD EARLAM

November 1995

This book is dedicated to Ian Haywood

Acknowledgments for illustrations

We would like to thank the following for permission to reproduce photographs: the American College of Surgeons' committee on trauma for photographs from the Advanced Trauma Life Support™ slide set; the Department of Education and Medical Illustration Services, St Bartholomew's Hospital; the Department of Medical Illustration, Hope Hospital, Salford; and the Medical Illustration Department, Withington Hospital, Manchester.

The line drawings were originally prepared by the Department of Education and Medical Illustration Services, St Bartholomew's Hospital; colour has been added and revisions done by Oxford Illustrators.

1 INITIAL ASSESSMENT AND MANAGEMENT— I: PRIMARY SURVEY

Peter Driscoll, David Skinner

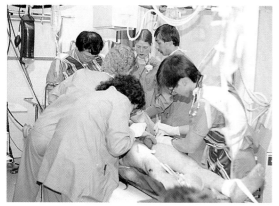

Trauma team in action.

Over 90% of the injured patients seen in British accident and emergency departments have been subjected to blunt trauma. These people are often difficult to assess because many of their injuries are hidden and therefore should be managed by a team approach using a predetermined plan for the initial assessment and urgent resuscitation. It is also important that each member of the team is familiar with their own role and those of their colleagues. These two essential elements will enable the members of the team to carry out their individual tasks simultaneously.

Objectives of the trauma team

- Identify and correct life threatening injuries
- Resuscitate the patient and stabilise the vital signs
- Determine the nature and extent of other injuries
- Categorise the injuries in order of priority
- Prepare and transport the patient to a place of definitive care

---

The trauma team
Personnel—The trauma team should initially comprise four doctors, five nurses, and a radiographer.
Team members' roles—Examples of paired roles and tasks are given on p 2. but assignments may vary among units depending on the resources available. To avoid chaos and disorganisation, there should be no more than six people physically touching the patient. The other team members must keep well back.

Before the patient arrives

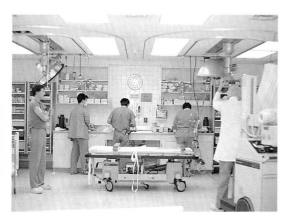

Many accident departments are warned by the ambulance service of the impending arrival of a seriously injured patient. This communication system can also provide the trauma team with essential information that can be acted on. Without it, the team has to wait until the prehospital personnel arrive at the department with the patient.

After the warning, the team should assemble in the resuscitation room and put on protective clothing. The absolute minimum is rubber latex gloves, plastic aprons, and eye protection because all blood and body fluids should be assumed to carry HIV and hepatitis viruses. Ideally, full protective clothing should be taken by each member of the team, and all must have been immunised against tetanus and the hepatitis B virus. Trauma patients often have sharp objects such as glass and other debris in their clothing, hair, and on their skin. Ordinary surgical gloves give no protection against this, so the people who undress the patient should initially wear more robust gloves.

While protective clothing is being put on, the team leaders should brief the team, ensuring that each member knows the task for which they are responsible. A final check of the equipment by the appropriate team members can then be made. As the resuscitation room must be kept fully stocked and ready for use at any time, only minimum preparation should be necessary.

Medical	Nursing and other staff
Team leader	• Coordinates the nursing team
• Coordinates the medical team	• Records clinical findings, laboratory results,
• Assesses the patient's chest, and depending on the skill of the rest of the team members, carries out particular procedures, such as pericardiocentesis and thoracotomy	intravenous and drug infusion, and the vital signs as called out by the circulation nurse
• Assimilates information and lists the investigations and treatment in order of priority	• Prepares sterile packs for procedures
• Liaises with other specialist personnel and questions the ambulance staff to ascertain the mechanism of injury, the prehospital findings, and the treatment given so far	• Assists the circulation nurses and brings extra equipment as necessary
Airway personnel	• Assists in securing the airway and stabilising the cervical spine
• Clears and secures the airway while taking appropriate cervical spine precautions	• Establishes a rapport with the patient in the resuscitation room. Ideally all information should be fed through this nurse to the patient
• Inserts central and arterial lines if required	
Circulation personnel	• Assists in the removal of the patient's clothes
• Assists in the removal of the patient's clothes	• Assists with starting intravenous infusions, chest drain insertion, and catheterisation. Monitors the fluid balance
• Establishes peripheral intravenous infusions and takes blood samples for investigations	
• Carries out certain procedures such as chest drain insertion, urinary catheterisation, and splinting	• Assists in special procedures such as thoracotomies
• Carries out other procedures depending on their skill level	• Measures the vital signs and connects the patient to the monitors
	Relatives' Nurse
	• Cares for the patient's relatives
	Radiographer
	• Takes three standard x ray films on all patients subjected to blunt trauma—chest, pelvis, and lateral cervical spine. A more selective approach is used with victims of penetrating trauma

Reception and transfer

(see Chapter 8)

Essential prehospital information

• Nature of the incident
• Number, age, and sex of the casualties
• The patient's complaints, priorities, and injuries
• Airway, ventilatory, and circulatory status
• The conscious level
• The management plan and its effect
• Estimated time of arrival

Those in charge of the airway should assess the patient in the back of the ambulance if there is a long distance between the ambulance bay and the resuscitation room. Provided there is no urgent airway problem requiring immediate intervention, the patient can be moved. Once the patient arrives in the resuscitation room, the nursing team leader should start the stop clock so that accurate times can be taken.

The transfer of the patient from the stretcher to the trolley must be coordinated so that there is no rotation of the spinal column or exacerbation of pre-existing injuries (see Chapter 8). Team members should also check that lines and leads are free so that they do not become disconnected or snagged.

PRIMARY SURVEY AND RESUSCITATION

Primary survey and resuscitation

Airway and cervical spine control
Breathing
Circulation and haemorrhage control
Dysfunction of the central nervous system
Exposure and environmental control

Secondary survey

Definitive care

The objectives of this phase are to hunt out and treat any immediately life threatening condition. Each patient should be assessed in the same way, with the appropriate tasks performed automatically and simultaneously by the team. It is vital that problems are anticipated and prepared for, rather than reacted to. If the patient deteriorates at any stage, the medical team leader must reassess the patient beginning again with the airway.

Airway management with protection of the cervical spine

As it is important to assume that the cervical spine has been damaged if there is suspicion of injury above the clavicles or if there is a history of a high speed impact, the doctor dealing with the airway should talk to the patient while the neck is kept manually in a neutral position by the airway nurse. If the patient replies in a normal voice, and gives logical answers to sensible questions, the airway is patent and the brain is being perfused adequately with oxygenated blood. If there is no

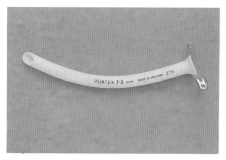

Guedel airway.

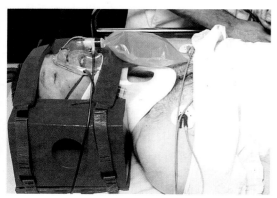

Nasopharyngeal airway.

Patient with rigid collar in place.

reply, the patient's mouth should be opened and any solid foreign objects removed with Magill forceps and fluid sucked out.

The complications of alcohol ingestion and possible injuries of the chest and abdomen increase the chance of the patient vomiting. If this starts, no attempt should be made to turn the patient's head to one side unless a cervical spine injury has been ruled out radiologically and clinically. If the patient is properly secured to a spinal (back) board, however, the whole body can be turned. In the absence of a spinal board the trolley should be tipped head down by 20° and the vomit sucked away with a rigid sucker as it appears in the mouth.

Chin lift or jaw thrust manoeuvres can be used to correct the position of the tongue which commonly obstructs the airway in unconscious patients. Those who have a gag reflex can maintain their own airway. The use of Guedel airways in these patients can precipitate vomiting, cervical movement, and a rise in intracranial pressure, so a nasopharyngeal airway is preferred provided that there is no evidence of a base of skull fracture.

If the patient is apnoeic, ventilation with a bag-valve-mask device may lead to gastric distension with air and can induce vomiting. Therefore patients without a gag reflex should be intubated so that ventilation can be carried out safely. Orotracheal intubation with in line stabilisation of the neck is recommended, rather than nasotracheal intubation. If this proves impossible then a surgical airway must be provided.

Once the airway has been cleared and secured, every patient should receive 100% oxygen at a flow rate of 15 l minute. The neck must then be examined quickly for wounds, tracheal position, venous distension, surgical emphysema, and laryngeal crepitus. Consideration can now be given to securing the cervical spine so that the airway nurse can safely release the patient's head and neck. This is done with either a semirigid collar, sand bags and tape, or a commercially available spine support. The only exception to this rule is the restless and thrashing patient. In this case, the cervical spine can be damaged by immobilising the head and neck while allowing the rest of the patient's body to move. A suboptimal level of immobilisation is therefore accepted, comprising a semirigid collar alone.

Common causes of inadequate ventilation

Bilateral:
Obstruction of the upper respiratory tract
Leak between the face and mask

Unilateral:
Intubation of the right main bronchus
Pneumothorax
Haemothorax
Foreign body in a main bronchi
Significant lung contusion

Immediately life threatening thoracic conditions

- Airway obstruction
- Tension pneumothorax
- Cardiac tamponade
- Open chest wound
- Massive haemothorax
- Flail chest

Breathing

The box opposite lists the six immediately life threatening thoracic conditions which must be urgently identified, and treated, during the primary survey and resuscitation phase (see Chapter 4).

To see if any of these conditions is present, all the clothes covering the front and sides of the chest must be removed. The respiratory rate, effort, and symmetry should then be recorded because these are sensitive indicators of underlying pulmonary contusion, haemothorax, pneumothorax, and fractured ribs. At the same time, the medical team leader should visually examine both sides of the chest for bruising, abrasions, open wounds, and evidence of penetrating trauma. Cardiac tamponade after trauma is usually associated with a penetrating injury. The team leader should also remember that because of intercostal muscle spasm, paradoxical breathing is seen with a flail chest only if the segment is large, or central, or when the patient's muscles become fatigued. The patient with a flail chest usually has a rapid, shallow, symmetrical, respiratory pattern initially.

After inspection, the chest should be auscultated and percussed to assess symmetry of ventilation and resonance. As listening over the anterior chest detects mainly air movement in the large airways, it is recommended that the medical team leader also listens over the axillas to gain a more accurate assessment of pulmonary ventilation. In this way a tension pneumothorax or a massive haemothorax can be identified. A tension pneumothorax should be relieved immediately by needle thoracocentesis and insection of a chest drain. A pneumothorax or haemothorax should be treated by inserting a chest drain with a gauge of >28 in the fifth intercostal space just anterior to the mid-axillary line. This enables air and fluid to be drained but should always be preceded by an intravenous line. During examination of the chest the patient should be attached to a pulse oximeter.

Circulation and haemorrhage control

Having assessed the patient's breathing, the medical team leader should look for any clinical signs of shock (see Chapter 5). Up to a 30% loss of blood volume will produce a tachycardia and reduced pulse pressure, but the blood pressure may remain within normal limits. There will be a consistent fall in the systolic blood pressure only when more than 30% of the blood volume has been lost. A urine output of less than 50 ml/hour in an adult indicates poor renal perfusion, which suggests poor perfusion of the tissues in general.

While the assessment is in progress, the circulation doctor must control any major external haemorrhage by direct pressure. In addition, provided that there are no contraindications, the pneumatic antishock garment should be considered in shocked patients who are suspected of having fractures of the pelvis. Tourniquets are used only when the affected limb is deemed unsalvageable.

Two wide bore (gauge 14–16) peripheral lines must then be inserted, preferably in the antecubital fossa. If this is impossible then venous access should be gained by either a venous cutdown or by inserting a short, wide bore, central line into the femoral or subclavian vein. If a subclavian approach is used and a chest drain is already in place then the central line must be inserted on the same side. As central vein cannulation can cause serious injury, this should be carried out only by experienced personnel.

Once the first cannula is in position 20 ml of blood should be drawn for group, type, or full cross match, full blood count, and measurement of urea and electrolyte concentrations. An arterial sample should also be taken for blood gas and pH analysis, but this can wait until the end of the primary survey. While venous access is being gained one of the circulation nurses must measure the blood pressure and record the rate, volume, and regularity of the pulse. An automatic blood pressure recorder and ECG monitor should also be attached to the patient.

In the UK, departmental policies vary as to the type of fluid initially given to injured patients to maintain the fluid balance. Some will start with colloid while others use Ringer's lactate (Hartmann's solution). It is therefore important that the local policy is known by the team leaders. A litre of colloid (or 2 l Ringer's lactate) must be given rapidly if the patient is hypovolaemic, and the signs reassessed. When there has been a limited response to the fluid bolus, or after a major injury, blood is required. To reduce the incidence of hypothermia, all fluids must be warmed before use.

In reassessing the circulatory state one of three responses may be seen:

(1) The vital signs return to normal after infusion of less than 1 l of colloid solution (or 2 l of Ringer's lactate). In such cases patients have lost less than 20% of their blood volume and are not actively bleeding.

(2) The vital signs initially improve with the infusion but then deteriorate. These patients are actively bleeding and have usually lost more than 20% of their blood volume. They require transfusion with typed blood and the source of the bleeding must be controlled. This often requires an operation.

(3) The vital signs do not improve at all. This suggests either that the shock has not been caused by hypovolaemia or that the patient is bleeding faster than blood is being infused. History, mechanism of injury, and the physical findings will help to distinguish between these two possibilities. Measurement of the central venous pressure and, in particular, its change after a fluid bolus may assist in diagnosis.

Patients with hypovolaemia whose vital signs do not improve at all have lost over 40% of their blood volume. The source of the bleeding is usually in the thorax, abdomen, or pelvis, and requires immediate operation.

Signs of shock

↑ Respiratory rate	↑ Skin pallid and clammy
↑ Heart rate	↑ Capillary refill time
↓ Blood pressure	↓ Urine output
↓ Pulse pressure	↓ Conscious level

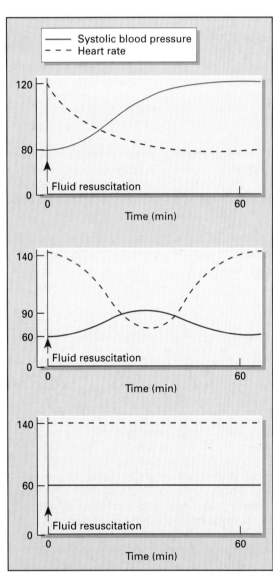

Line diagrams showing the three responses to fluid resuscitation.

Conscious level can be assessed by the ATLS system of AVPU[m]:

A = **A**lert
V = Reports to **v**oice
P = Responds to **p**ain
U = **U**nconscious

Dysfunction of the central nervous system

A rapid assessment of brain and spinal cord function is made by assessing the pupillary reflexes and by asking patients to "put out your tongue", "wiggle your toes", and "squeeze my fingers". Remember, however, that these quick manoeuvres will detect only gross neurological damage. A more detailed assessment, including assessment of the Glasgow coma scale, can be used if there is time, but it is often delayed until the secondary survey.

Exposure

By this stage, all clothing necessary to perform the primary survey should have been cut away with large sharp scissors so that the patient has been moved as little as possible. The remainder should now be removed. To prevent patients subsequently becoming cold, they should be covered with warm blankets when not being examined, and the resuscitation room should be kept warm.

By the end of the primary survey the medical team leader must make sure that all the allocated tasks have been completed. In addition, the vital signs should continue to be recorded every five minutes so that the patient's progress or deterioration can be detected. Only when all the ventilatory and circulatory problems have been corrected can the team continue with the more detailed secondary survey. As the primary survey and resuscitation phase is underway, the relatives' nurse should greet any of the patient's friends or relatives who arrive. She can then take them to a private room which has all necessary facilities and stay there, providing support and information. Relatives should not be prevented from seeing the patient in the resuscitation room. However, they must be accompanied by the relatives' nurse so that they can receive a full explanation on what is going on (see chapter 16).

2 INITIAL ASSESSMENT AND MANAGEMENT— II: SECONDARY SURVEY

Objectives of secondary survey

- Examine the patient from head to toe and front to back
- Take a complete medical history
- Assimilate all clinical, laboratory and radiological information
- Formulate a management plan for the patient

The objectives of this phase are listed opposite. In addition, it should be standard practice to do lateral cervical spine, chest, and pelvic radiography in patients with blunt trauma. Protective lead aprons must therefore be worn by those staff who continue to manage the patient. One doctor, who may be the team leader, should ensure that the secondary survey is orderly and complete.

Head

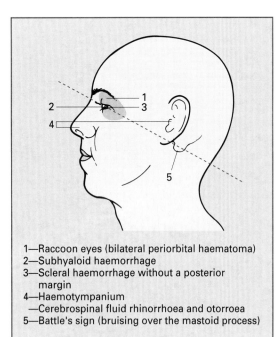

1—Raccoon eyes (bilateral periorbital haematoma)
2—Subhyaloid haemorrhage
3—Scleral haemorrhage without a posterior margin
4—Haemotympanium
 —Cerebrospinal fluid rhinorrhoea and otorroea
5—Battle's sign (bruising over the mastoid process)

Signs of a base of skull fracture.

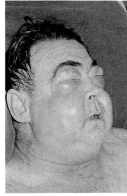

Extreme facial oedema.

Scalp

This must be examined for lacerations, swellings, or depressions. Its entire surface must be inspected and palpated but the occiput will have to wait until the patient is turned. Visual inspection may discover fractures in the base of the lacerations, but wounds should not be probed blindly as further damage to underlying structures can result. If there is major bleeding from the scalp, digital pressure or a self-retaining retractor should be used.

Neurological state

A "mini-neurological" examination of the patient can now be carried out. This comprises an assessment of the conscious level using the Glasgow coma scale, the pupillary response, and the presence of any lateralising signs (see Chapter 6). One of the circulation nurses should continue to monitor these variables. If there is any deterioration hypoxia or hypovolaemia must be ruled out before considering intracranial injury.

Base of skull

Externally the base of the skull runs from the mastoid process to the orbit, so fractures of the base of the skull may produce signs along this line. When there is cerebrospinal fluid rhinorrhoea or otorrhoea, the fluid is invariably mixed with blood which will delay the clotting of the blood and produce a double ring pattern if dropped on to a sheet. Examination with an auroscope may precipitate meningitis in patients with such problems and is therefore contraindicated.

Eyes

These must be examined early, before orbital swelling may make it impossible. Haemorrhages inside or outside the globe, foreign bodies under the lids, and evidence of penetrating injury must be noted. Visual acuity can be tested rapidly by asking the patient to read a label. If the patient is unconscious the corneal reflex should be assessed.

Face

The face should be palpated symmetrically for deformities and tenderness. Loose or lost teeth must also be identified. Instability of the maxilla can be assessed by traction on the upper incisors and, if it is unstable, suggests a middle third fracture of the facial skeleton. Though these may be associated with fractures of the base of the skull, only those that are compromising the airway need to be treated immediately. This usually entails pulling the fractured facial segment forwards to clear the airway. Mandibular fractures can also cause airway obstruction because of the loss of stability of the tongue. In these cases a traction suture is inserted into the tongue and the ends taped to the face or chest (see Chapter 7).

Neck

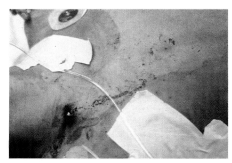
Gunshot wound of the neck.

With the head held firmly by an assistant, the cervical immobilisation devices can be removed and the neck re-examined. Once the features described previously have been reassessed, the cervical spinous processes should be palpated for tenderness and deformities. The posterior cervical neck muscles should also be palpated for spasm and tenderness. Conscious patients will also assist by telling if there is any pain in the neck and, if so, its location.

Lacerations must be inspected, but if a wound penetrates platysma it should be explored under general anaesthesia in the operating room.

A lateral cervical spine radiograph showing all seven cervical vertebrae and the cervicothoracic junction is essential in patients with multiple injuries. Nevertheless, this can still miss 15% of fractures, so an anteroposterior radiograph and odontoid peg views are required for full evaluation of the cervical spine. This can be delayed until the secondary survey has been completed.

Thorax

Potentially life threatening thoracic conditions

- Pulmonary contusion
- Cardiac contusion
- Ruptured diaphragm
- Aortic tear
- Oesophageal rupture
- Airway obstruction

The priority at this stage is to identify conditions that are potentially life threatening. In most cases this will require specialist investigation to confirm the team leader's initial suspicions, arising from the mechanism of injury and the clinical findings.

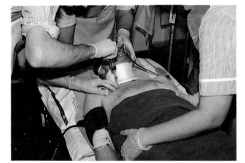
Needle aspiration of a pneumothorax.

Pulmonary and cardiac contusions are potentially life threatening and should be considered when the chest wall has received a severe direct blow. Cardiac arrhythmias or an infarct pattern on the ECG may reflect cardiac contusion. The thoracic aorta can be torn when the patient has been subjected to a rapid deceleration force such as a road traffic accident or a fall from a height. A high index of suspicion, together with a thorough examination and a chest x ray film taken in the erect position are essential in these cases (see Chapter 4). Ruptured diaphragm and perforated oesophagus can follow both blunt and penetrating trauma, and diagnosis is usually dependent on the appearance in the chest radiograph.

The chest wall must be re-inspected for bruising, signs of obstruction, asymmetry of movement, and wounds. Acceleration and deceleration forces can produce extensive thoracic injuries; these invariably leave marks on the chest wall which should lead the team to consider the particular types of injury. For example, the bruise resulting from pressure exerted by a diagonal seat belt may overlay a fractured clavicle, a thoracic aortic tear, pulmonary contusion, or pancreatic laceration. The mark caused by impact with the steering wheel suggests a sternal fracture with cardiac contusion.

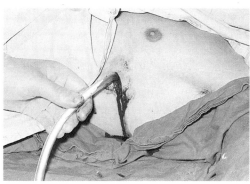
Chest drain in situ.

The clinician should then palpate the chest by feeling the ribs in the apices of both axillas and then continue in a caudal manner. The presence of any crepitus, tenderness, and subcutaneous emphysema must be noted. Attention can then be directed to the anterior aspect of the chest by pressing on both clavicles, each rib, and the sternum. Palpation is completed by squeezing the chest in a lateral and anteroposterior plane to detect the presence of multiple rib fractures. Auscultation and percussion of the whole chest can then be carried out to check for asymmetry.

Abdomen

Signs of urethral injury

- Blood at external urethral meatus
- Bruising of scrotum or perineum
- High riding prostate

Rectal examination

- Sphincter tone
- Presence of rectal damage
- Presence of pelvic fractures
- Prostate position
- Blood in the faecal residue

Signs of renal injury

- Flank pain
- Flank mass
- Flank bruising
- Haematuria

Indications of positive diagnostic peritoneal lavage

- >5 ml free blood aspirated from the peritoneal cavity
- Enteric contents aspirated from the peritoneal cavity
- Lavage fluid leaking into the chest drains or urinary catheter

In the lavage fluid
- >100 000 red blood cells × 10^9/l
- Bile
- Food products
- Bacteria

The team leader's aim in examining the abdomen is simply to decide if the patient requires a laparotomy. A precise diagnosis of which particular viscus has been injured is both time consuming and of little relevance at this stage.

A thorough examination of the whole abdomen is required, so the pelvis and the perineum must be assessed. All bruising, abnormal movement, signs of male urethral injury, and wounds must be noted. Any exposed bowel should be covered with warm, saline-soaked swabs. Lacerations can then be inspected but not probed blindly as further damage may result. If a laceration extends into muscle, specialist advice is necessary as further investigations, including laparotomy, may be required (see Chapter 9).

The abdomen must then be palpated and any signs of tenderness recorded. As squeezing the pelvis in two planes will detect only severe abnormalities, all patients with blunt trauma must undergo pelvic radiography. Finally, a rectal examination must be carried out.

A catheter should be inserted so that the patient's rate of urine output can be measured. A perurethral approach can be used if there is is no evidence of urethral injury. If an injury is suspected, however, a suprapubic catheter should be inserted and subsequently a retrograde urethrogram will be required. Irrespective of the catheterisation procedure, the urine must be tested for blood. A positive result supports the diagnosis of a renal injury and further investigations are required. A one shot intravenous pyelogram can be taken in the resuscitation room and this will show if both kidneys are present, functioning and with, or without, major disruption. This rapid investigation is commonly reserved for patients who require an urgent operation but in whom the presence of any major renal disease must be excluded. If there is no urgency, a definitive intravenous pyelogram and cystogram may be carried out at the end of the secondary survey. Urine should be saved for possible future microscopic examination and analysis of drug concentrations.

Pronounced gastric distension is common in crying children, adults with head or abdominal injuries, and patients who have been ventilated with a bag and mask. The insertion of a gastric tube decompresses the stomach, reduces the risks of aspiration, and facilitates the abdominal examination of these patients.

An intra-abdominal bleed should be suspected if there are fractures of the ribs overlying the liver and spleen (5–11), the patient is haemodynamically unstable, or there are marks caused by seat belts or tyres over the abdomen. The detection of abdominal tenderness may be unreliable, however, particularly in patients with sensory defects caused by neurological damage or drugs, or if there are fractures of the lower ribs or pelvis. In these cases, diagnostic peritoneal lavage should be carried out to help rule out an intraperitoneal injury. Ideally this should be done by, or in the presence of, the general surgeon who will be responsible for any subsequent laparotomy.

Extremities

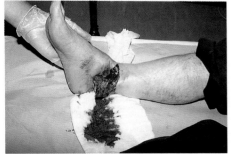

Open fracture and dislocation of the right ankle.

All the limbs must be inspected for bruising, wounds, and deformities, and examined for vascular and neurological defects. The viability of the skin overlying fractures or dislocations must also be assessed before and after the deformity has been corrected. This reduction should be carried out before radiography if the blood supply to the surrounding skin and soft tissues is compromised. Crepitus and instability can then be assessed by palpating and rotating all long bones. The level of active and passive movement must also be recorded. The examiner must palpate all the bones in the limbs: metacarpal, metatarsal, and phalangeal fractures can easily be overlooked and may result in subsequent severe disability if left untreated.

Swabs should be taken for microbiological analysis from sites of open fractures. The wounds can then be covered with sterile dressings. Splinting of broken limbs is important because it reduces further damage to soft tissues, pain, and possibly the production of fat emboli. A Polaroid picture taken before covering an open fracture will prevent repeated inspection and reduce the risk of infection.

Spinal column

A detailed neurological examination needs to be carried out at this stage to find out if there are any abnormalities in the peripheral nervous system. Sensory and motor defects, and evidence of priaprism, can help indicate the level and extent of the spinal injury. If the cord has been transected above the level of the sympathetic outflow, neurogenic shock results. This is manifested by hypotension without a corresponding tachycardia. The blood pressure falls as a consequence of vasodilatation but its extent depends on how much sympathetic tone remains. For example, transection of the cervical spinal cord removes all vasoconstrictor tone and results in profound hypotension.

If a spinal injury is suspected, the patient should be moved only by a well coordinated "log rolling" technique. As the patient is turned away from the examiner, debris can be cleared away and the back examined from occiput to heels. Bruising and open wounds must be noted and the chest auscultated. The examiner's fingers should then palpate each spinous process in turn, so that any deformity or tenderness (in the conscious patient) can be detected. The paraspinal muscles are then similarly assessed. Finally the buttock cheeks must be separated so that any exit or entry wounds in this area are discovered. The patient can then be "log rolled" back into the supine position. In addition, the nursing team leader should make an initial assessment of the skin using a pressure sore scoring system – for example, the Waterlow system. In elderly people and other high risk patients meticulous care must be taken to prevent the development of pressure sores.

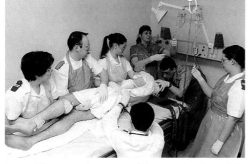

Log rolling a patient to enable examination of the back.

Patients can have vertebral column injuries without the presence of physical signs on examination

Soft tissue injuries

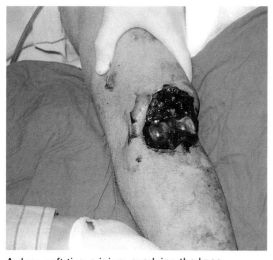

A deep soft tissue injury overlying the knee.

A detailed inspection of the whole of the patient's skin is needed to find out the number and extent of the soft tissue injuries. Each breach in the skin should be inspected to ascertain its site, depth, and the presence of any underlying structural damage which will require surgical repair during the definitive care phase. Once the patient is stable, however, superficial wounds can be cleaned, irrigated, and dressed.

Medical history

This should be completed now. Information may be available from the patient, relatives, and ambulance crew. A useful mnemonic is given in the box. It is crucial to find out the mechanism of the injury as this gives invaluable information about the forces the patient was subjected to and the direction of impact. Further help will come from a description of the damage to the car or details of the weapon used (see Chapter 20).

REASSESSMENT

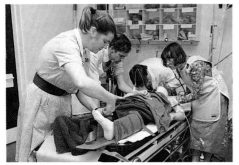

Trauma team in action during the secondary survey.

The team leader must constantly re-evaluate the response to resuscitation:

(1) Is the patient improving, deteriorating, or unchanged since resuscitation started? If the patient is not improving then the **A**irway, **B**reathing, **C**irculation, and **D**isability must be reassessed. As the patient's condition can change rapidly, repeated examination and constant monitoring are essential.

(2) What is the extent of the injuries and what are the priorities for treatment?

(3) Has an injury been missed? After blunt trauma, if no injury has been found in an area of the body between two injured sites, then the patient must be re-examined. Blunt trauma tends not to "skip" regions.

(4) Has analgesia been given? Victims of major trauma require pain relief. A mixture of 50% nitrous oxide and 50% oxygen (Entonox) may be given until the secondary survey has been completed. Morphine can then be given intravenously, the dose being titrated against the patient's response.

(5) What is the patient's tetanus status and are antibiotics required?

(6) Are any further radiological investigations required? This depends on the condition of the patient. If he or she is hypoxic or haemodynamically unstable then these problems must be dealt with first. Once the condition stabilises, radiographs of particular sites of injury can be taken along with other specialised investigations. It is an important part of the team leader's responsibilities to assess the priorities of these investigations. Furthermore, adequate resuscitation equipment and monitors must be immediately available in the places where these radiographs are taken.

The medical team leader is responsible for all documentation, which must be accurate and complete. If a criminal cause for the injury is suspected all clothes, loose debris, bullets, and shrapnel must be collected, labelled, placed in waxed bags, and signed for before they are released to the appropriate authorities according to locally established policy.

Responsibility for continuing care should be formally handed over, usually to the duty senior intensive care physician or surgeon, when the patient leaves the accident and emergency department. Nevertheless the same level of care carried out in the resuscitation room must be maintained during the patient's transfer to the ward, theatre, or specialist centre (see Chapter 21). Finally, the nurse dealing with the patient's relatives and friends must inform them about the transfer. When the patient is to be moved to another hospital, this nurse should also help them to make their own transportation arrangements.

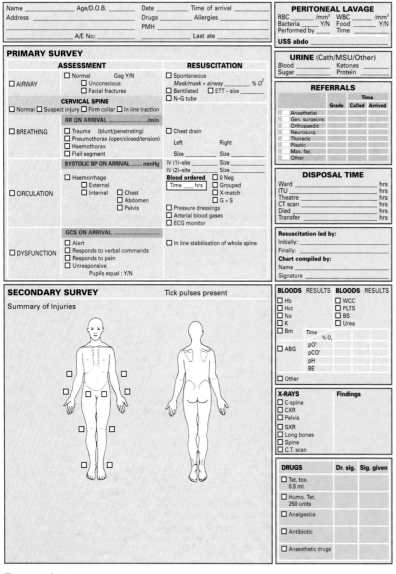

Trauma sheet.

3 THE UPPER AIRWAY

David Watson

First vital minutes

Signs and symptoms of upper airway obstruction

- Noisy breathing
- Effort of breathing: tracheal tugging; intercostal recession; abdominal see-saw movement
- Increased use of accessory muscles
- Apnoea (late)
- Cyanosis (late)

Indications for securing an airway with an endotracheal tube

- Apnoea
- Obstruction of upper airway
- Protection of lower airway from soiling with blood or vomitus
- Respiratory insufficiency
- Impending or potential compromise of airway (prophylactic intubation)—for example, after facial burns or continuous seizures after intravenous diazepam
- Raised intracranial pressure requiring hyperventilation

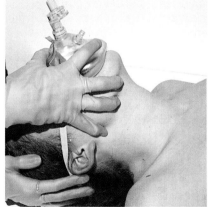

Mouth-to-face mask.

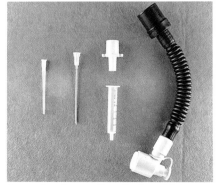

Apparatus for needle cricothyroidotomy. Modified large bore intravenous cannula and anaesthetic connections.

All severely injured patients have hypoxaemia in varying degrees. As soon as medical help arrives the first priority must be to ensure that the patient's airway is clear and ventilation is unimpaired. Immediate administration of supplementary oxygen to the unobstructed airway is of paramount importance. Remember that in the first vital minutes the cervical spine of any patient with trauma should be considered broken until proved otherwise. The neck must be kept stabilised without traction (for example, by using a spinal board, sand bags, and a hard collar) at all times until the possibility of neck injury is excluded.

In an unconscious patient any obstruction to the airway must be removed under direct vision. The laryngeal and pharyngeal reflexes should then be assessed and respiratory performance examined. If protective reflexes are adequate—for example, the patient is coughing—retracting the tongue forward by employing the chin lift or jaw thrust manoeuvre or inserting an anaesthetic type airway or nasopharyngeal tube may suffice. If the reflexes are depressed or absent—that is, there is no gag reflex when oropharyngeal suction is attempted in an unconscious patient—the airway must be secured at the earliest opportunity by intubation with an appropriately sized endotracheal tube with a low pressure cuff.

Patients with hypoxia or apnoea must be ventilated and oxygenated before intubation is attempted. Ventilation can be achieved with a mouth-to-face mask or bag-valve-face mask. Studies suggest that ventilation techniques with a bag-valve-face mask are less effective when performed by one person rather than two people, when one of the pair can use both hands to assure a good seal. When only one person is present to provide ventilation the method employing the mouth-to-face mask is preferred. During such manoeuvres the neck must be kept immobilised.

If intubation is performed a large bore gastric tube should also be passed. Nasal passage of a gastric tube is contraindicated in patients with suspected basal skull fractures or injury to the cribriform plate.

Tracheostomy is rarely necessary as an emergency procedure. Severe distorting injury to the structures above or at the level of the larynx can render endotracheal intubation impossible, but cricothyroidotomy—for example, with a large bore intravenous cannula—is preferred to emergency tracheostomy in such circumstances.

In patients with fractured ribs with or without a pneumothorax chest drainage on the side of the fractures is mandatory before artificial ventilation is undertaken. A tension pneumothorax should always be suspected when a patient with a recent crush injury has obvious respiratory distress or cyanosis. In patients with a chest injury complicated by pneumothorax an apical chest drain should be inserted through the space between the fifth and sixth ribs, just anterior to the mid-axillary line. If there is blood in the pleural cavity an additional basal drain may be required.

An open pneumothorax should be managed initially by inserting a chest tube to relieve any accumulated air and prevent the development of a tension pneumothorax. The opening can then be closed temporarily with either a petroleum jelly gauze or other non-porous dressing.

Indications for oxygenation and ventilation

- Ventilatory assistance is required when there is excessive respiratory work or obvious ventilatory insufficiency
- Failure of adequate oxygenation (PaO_2 <9 kPa) when the patient is breathing a high inspired oxygen concentration (6 l/min O_2 by facemask) demands endotracheal intubation and assisted positive pressure ventilation

Once the airway is secured the adequacy of the exchange of respiratory gases must be evaluated. The respiratory rate can be counted and respiratory effort assessed. Measurements of blood gas tensions should be undertaken as soon as is practicable.

Artificial ventilation in patients without respiratory failure must also be considered when there is coincidental head injury. Hypercapnia and hypoxaemia from asphyxia or inadequate ventilation with fluctuations in arterial blood pressure cause considerable deterioration in cerebral function. This is probably secondary to alterations in cerebral blood flow that adversely affect intracranial pressure.

Hospital management

Intubation of patients with head injuries

- Assume the patient has a cervical fracture
- An anaesthetist performs laryngoscopy while an assistant holds the patient's head
- Pressure on the cricoid must be provided by an assistant to prevent aspiration of gastric contents

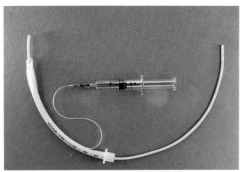

Gum elastic bougie and endotracheal tube.

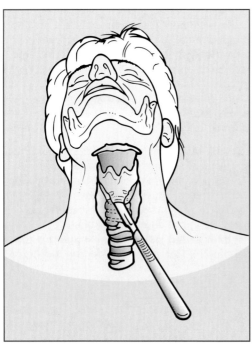

Cricothyroidotomy with scalpel.

An anaesthetist experienced in caring for victims of trauma should be available to examine the patient immediately on arrival at hospital. Evaluation of the patient's airway must proceed simultaneously with treatment. If the airway is satisfactory treatment may consist simply of increased oxygen delivery. If the airway is compromised or the patient needs ventilatory support a secure intratracheal airway, if not already in place, is required. Patients with hypoxia or apnoea must be ventilated and oxygenated before intubation is attempted.

The route of choice for securing the airway depends on several factors. Blunt trauma of the head and face is associated with an incidence of fractures of the cervical spine of 5 to 10%.[1] Patients with trauma should be assumed to have a cervical fracture until proved otherwise; manipulation of the neck is strictly contraindicated. Doctors in the United Kingdom generally accept that laryngoscopy and orotracheal intubation after induction of anaesthesia and muscle paralysis can be performed by a competent operator with minimal changes in the position of the cervical vertebrae while an assistant holds the patient's head. Although optimum exposure of the larynx is not achievable under such conditions, experienced anaesthetists can intubate patients without clearly visualising the vocal cords. This may require aids such as the gum elastic bougie. Pressure on the cricoid must be provided by a skilled assistant to protect the patient from aspirating gastric contents.[2] The stomach may already have been emptied as much as possible by the passage of a nasogastric tube with the neck immobilised. Alternatively, if the patient's condition permits, fibreoptic endoscopy may facilitate difficult orotracheal or nasotracheal intubation.

Surgical cricothyroidotomy may be necessary for patients who cannot be intubated either nasally or orally. Often these patients have massive facial trauma. Although surgical cricothyroidotomy can be performed through a small midline incision in the cricothyroid membrane, life saving oxygenation can also be provided by needle cricothyroidotomy with a cannula connected to wall oxygen at 15 l/minute with either a Y connector or a side hole in the tubing attached between the oxygen source and the cannula. Spontaneous respiration after needle cricothyroidotomy, however, can be extremely difficult, requiring large pressure changes in the airway and considerable ventilatory effort. Intermittent insufflation (for which sedation and muscle paralysis are necessary) can be achieved by occluding the open end of the Y connector or the side hole of the oxygen tubing. The patient can be ventilated by this technique for only 30–45 minutes which limits its usefulness particularly in those with head injuries. Jet insufflation must also be used with caution when obstruction by a foreign body is suspected in the glottic area.

Anaesthetic considerations

Anaesthetists caring for patients who are critically ill reduce the doses of all anaesthetics because hypovolaemia and hypotension alter the distribution and pharmacokinetics of drugs, thereby exaggerating their clinical effects. Opiates and barbiturates are therefore given in smaller doses to avoid cardiovascular depression. Ketamine and halogenated hydrocarbons such as halothane raise intracranial pressure and are contraindicated in trauma of the head. Ketamine (1 to 2 mg/kg) and partial opiate agonists such as nalbuphine, however, are useful in trauma that is complicated by haemorrhagic shock. Muscle relaxants given to facilitate intubation include suxamethonium (1.0 mg/kg), pancuronium (0.1 to 0.2 mg/kg), vecuronium (0.1 to 0.2 mg/kg) or atracurium (0.4 mg/kg). Often patients have taken drugs such as opiates, cocaine, and marijuana before suffering trauma. These may interact with anaesthetics. Ethanol enhances the effect of anaesthetics and sedatives and reduces the minimum alveolar concentration of volatile general anaesthetics required.[3]

Before embarking on intubation an anaesthetist will check the equipment, including the suction and oxygen delivery apparatus. Anaesthetics should be ready in labelled syringes, and duplicate ampoules should be easily accessible. Vasoactive drugs such as atropine should also be ready in syringes in case untoward bradycardia complicates extended laryngoscopy. A skilled assistant must be at hand to apply pressure on the cricoid. The neck must be kept stabilised. Secure venous access is mandatory. Ideally a pulse oximeter should be attached to the patient's earlobe or finger to give a continuous display of the arterial haemoglobin oxygen saturation.

Anaesthesia is induced with the best possible monitoring available and only after administration of oxygen. Pressure on the cricoid is maintained by the assistant. Neuromuscular blockade is produced by suxamethonium, and intubation proceeds with the onset of paralysis and relaxation of the jaw.

Patients with responsive airway reflexes require induction of anaesthesia and muscle paralysis for the airway to be secured by either an oral or a nasotracheal route. Deeply unconscious patients with trauma of the head and brain injury should not be intubated without prior administration of a cerebral sedative and muscle relaxant, hence avoiding dangerous increases in cerebral blood volume and intracranial pressure during laryngoscopy. Nasotracheal intubation should not be undertaken if fractures of the base of the skull or of the cribriform plate are suspected.

Drugs contraindicated in trauma

Head injuries
- Ketamine increases intracranial pressure
- Halothane and enflurane increase intracranial pressure

Burns and spinal cord injuries
- Suxamethonium is safe during the first 24 hours but subsequently it can cause potentially lethal hyperkalaemia

Eye injuries
- Suxamethonium is relatively contraindicated as it raises intraocular pressure

---

Essential equipment for endotracheal intubation

- Laryngoscope
- Endotracheal tube
- Connections
- Inflating bag (such as Ambu bag)
- 10 ml Syringe for cuff inflation
- Suction apparatus
- Bougie or introducer catheter
- Magill curved forceps

Intubation technique

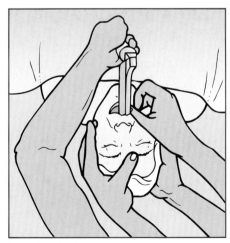

Inserting the laryngoscope.

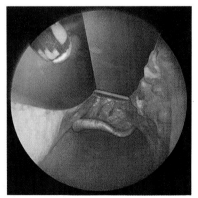

Lifting the root of the tongue.

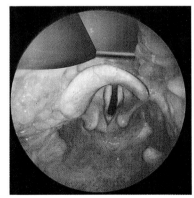

Direct visualisation of the glottis.

The anaesthetist takes the laryngoscope in his or her left hand and inserts it into the right hand side of the patient's mouth, thereby moving the tongue to the left. While carefully observing the back of the tongue he or she advances the curved blade of the laryngoscope until the epiglottis comes into view.

The upper airway

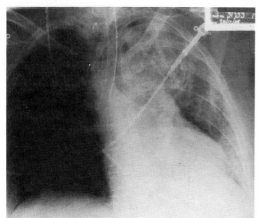

Chest radiograph showing inadvertent intubation of the right main bronchus.

The tip of the blade is moved anterior to the epiglottis and the whole lower jaw lifted upwards, taking care not to move the neck. This should expose the arytenoid cartilages and vocal cords. The tracheal rings should be visible beyond. Under direct vision the anaesthetist advances a 60 cm gum elastic bougie or the endotracheal tube, aiming for the left vocal cord. If a gum elastic bougie is used a cut cuffed endotracheal tube of the appropriate size is subsequently "rail roaded" into the trachea. A size 8 tube is usually suitable for women and a size 9 for men. The cuff of the endotracheal tube is then inflated with air from a syringe until an airtight seal is secured. The chest should be auscultated in both axillas to exclude intubation of the right main bronchus or oesophagus. An end tidal carbon dioxide monitor attached to the endotracheal tube between the adaptor and the ventilator device will rapidly confirm that the endotracheal tube is in the trachea. Pressure on the cricoid can only now be released and the tube secured with tapes.

After intubation ventilation should proceed with a tidal volume of about 10 ml/kg at a rate of about 10 breaths each minute. Although capnography and pulse oximetry may provide immediate non-invasive assessment of oxygenation and the adequacy of ventilation, the arterial blood gas tensions should be analysed at the first opportunity. Radiography of the chest should also be performed routinely after endotracheal intubation to catalogue the position of the endotracheal tube in the bronchial tree.

In conclusion, providing oxygen and ventilatory support as early as possible are prerequisites for successful resuscitation in victims of major trauma. Otherwise, as Haldane observed, hypoxia not only stops the machine but wrecks the machinery.

Illustrations of the technique of intubation were reproduced from *A Systematic Guide to Intubation* (by P Lotz, F W Annefeld, and W K Hirlinger) by kind permission of the publisher, Atelier Flad, Eckental, West Germany.

1 McCabe JB, Angelos MG. Injury to the head and face in patients with cervical spine injury. *Am J Emerg Med* 1984;**2**:333.
2 Sellick BA. Cricoid pressure to control regurgitation of stomach contents during induction of anaesthesia. *Lancet* 1961;**ii**:404.
3 Bruce DL. Alcoholism and anesthesia. *Anesth Analg* 1983;**62**:84.

4 CHEST INJURIES

Stephen Rooney, Stephen Westaby, Timothy Graham

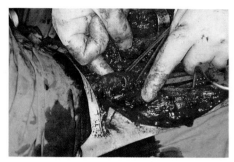

Stab wounds in the thoracic inlet. Exposure of the transsected trachea and oesophagus by median sternotomy.

Chest injuries are responsible for 25% of trauma deaths in the United Kingdom. Many patients who sustain major intrathoracic injuries die at the site of the accident. Those who reach hospital are therefore a self selected group, most of whom should survive with early and appropriate management. Less than 15% will require surgery; the remainder can be managed by simple measures such as intercostal drainage, adequate analgesia, careful fluid management, and regular physiotherapy. Failure to manage this group of patients properly may cause death, possibly during surgery for extra-thoracic injuries.

These thoracic injuries should not be underestimated. They may result in reduced cardiac output or respiratory impairment or, as is most often the case, a combination of the two. Blood loss, ventilatory failure, lung contusion or collapse, and displacement of mediastinal structures may cause hypoxia and acidosis which rapidly compound the adverse effects of other injuries. The aim of early intervention and resuscitation is to restore adequate delivery of oxygen to the tissues. Successful management of thoracic trauma is dependent therefore on effective cardiopulmonary resuscitation followed by the detection and rapid treatment of immediately life threatening injuries.

As major intrathoracic injuries may occur without chest wall damage, other more obvious injuries may delay the diagnosis of chest trauma. Diagnosis should depend on prediction and exclusion rather than direct manifestation of injury; the examination should be guided by a high index of suspicion for specific injuries. Distinct patterns of injury (high velocity, low velocity, crush, or penetrating trauma) are associated with differing thoracic and other injuries. In addition other predictors are associated with head and abdominal injuries; evidence of major haemorrhage in the absence of abdominal swelling or major bony injury; wounds, bruising, or seatbelt marks on the chest wall; and any degree of respiratory distress.

Type of injury

Chest wall injury	Possible intrathoracic injury	Common associated injuries
Penetrating injuries		
Defect in muscle layer at site of injury which may well have sealed itself	Laceration of heart, great vessels, oesophagus, or major airway	Lacerated liver or spleen
Crush injuries		
Rib fractures with or without flail segment	Ruptured bronchus, cardiac contusion, pulmonary contusion	Lacerated liver or spleen, thoracic spinal fractures
High velocity (deceleration) injuries		
Chest wall may be intact, or sternal fracture or rib fractures with or without flail segment	Aortic rupture, cardiac contusion, major airway injury, ruptured diaphragm	Head or facial injury, cervical spine injury, long bone fractures, lacerated liver or spleen
Low velocity (direct blow) injuries		
Sternal or rib fractures	Pulmonary, cardiac contusion	Lacerated liver or spleen

Chest injuries

Primary survey

ABC principle of resuscitation

- Establish a safe **A**irway
- Restore the mechanics of **B**reathing
- Maintain the **C**irculation

Pathophysiology of life threatening injuries

- *Tissue hypoxia* results from inadequate delivery of oxygen secondary to hypovolaemia (blood loss), ventilation/perfusion mismatch (lung contusion/collapse), and intrathoracic pressure changes (tension pneumothorax, open pneumothorax), or a combination of these (haemopneumothorax)
- *Acidosis* may be metabolic secondary to tissue hypoperfusion or respiratory. Respiratory acidosis may be caused by inadequate ventilation (airway injury or obstruction), intrathoracic pressure changes, and altered level of consciousness
- *Low cardiac output* may be secondary to loss of blood volume, cardiac tamponade, or metabolic derangement

During the primary survey management is begun and life-threatening injuries are identified simultaneously. Intervention is based on the immediate life threatening problem but follows the ABC principle of resuscitation.

Airway

The first priority is patency of the airway. This should be assessed by listening for air movement at the nose and mouth, and looking for movement of the intercostal and supraclavicular muscles. The oropharynx should be checked for foreign body obstruction. Impending hypoxia is indicated sometimes by subtle changes in the breathing pattern, which becomes more shallow and tachypnoeic. Cyanosis is often a late sign secondary to peripheral hypoperfusion and blood loss. Securing an airway can be difficult and hazardous in patients who have received injuries to the neck or upper chest.

Breathing

The patient's chest must be completely exposed so that the respiratory movement and quality of ventilation can be assessed by observation, palpation, and auscultation. The mechanics of breathing can be disrupted by major airway obstruction, haemothorax or pneumothorax, flail chest, pain, or pulmonary contusion.

Circulation

The pulse should be assessed for quality, rate, and regularity. The blood pressure and width of pulse pressure must be measured, as despite considerable blood loss a normal blood pressure can be maintained by vasoconstriction. The peripheral circulation is assessed by skin colour and temperature. Venous distension in the neck may not always be present in a hypovolaemic patient with cardiac tamponade. An electrocardiograph should always be attached to the patient.

Immediate thoracotomy for life threatening injuries

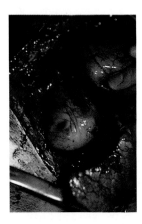

Immediate thoracotomy for blunt trauma with cardiac herniation. The severely contused heart was strangulated in the atrioventricular groove. The patient required an intra-aortic balloon pump for three days.

Immediate thoracotomy for life threatening injury

- Following injury when control of haemorrhage or tamponade is vital for resuscitation
- When there is EMD following penetrating chest injury
- For uncontrollable intra-abdominal haemorrhage to cross clamp the aorta and preferentially perfuse the brain and heart, and facilitate surgical control of the source of bleeding

An immediate thoracotomy is indicated on the basis of physical findings without investigations when closed cardiac massage for cardiac arrest or electromechanical dissociation is ineffective in a hypovolaemic patient. This may occur when resuscitation is impossible without control of haemorrhage or tamponade; when there is massive abdominal bleeding; or when there is myocardial electrical activity but no cardiac output following penetrating chest injury. Thoracotomy enables relief of tamponade, internal cardiac massage, and cross-clamping of the aorta, which will help to restore the perfusion pressure to the brain and coronary arteries while controlling intra-abdominal haemorrhage. This emergency surgery may take the form of median sternotomy, anterolateral thoracotomy, or lateral thoracotomy according to the nature of the injury, the surgeon's experience, and facilities available. Once the cardiac output to the upper body has been restored, the requirement for craniotomy must be determined quickly and before abdominal surgery is undertaken. In the presence of potentially lethal brain, cardiac, or aortic injury other injuries are of secondary importance.

Such an emergency thoracotomy is not indicated without a surgeon. Thoracotomy for blunt chest injury and cardiac arrest is rarely successful; most reports confirm that only patients with penetrating injuries benefit. Open chest surgery at the site of the accident is invariably unsuccessful.

Resuscitation

Intubation and positive pressure ventilation may be necessary to establish an airway and restore the mechanics of breathing. Once an adequate upper airway has been secured oxygen transport will be improved by maximising the inspired oxygen concentration. Early correction of hypoxia and acidosis is vital, particularly in the presence of head injury to prevent secondary brain damage or when further surgery is to be undertaken. This must be based on the knowledge of arterial blood gas tensions and acid-base analyses.

The amount of crystalloid fluid infused should be carefully considered. Initially 1 litre of Hartmann's/Ringer's solution should be infused as quickly as possible and the clinical response carefully monitored. During this time blood should be crossmatched and type specific Rhesus negative blood obtained if possible. Base deficit is a sensitive indicator of oxygen debt and changes in oxygen delivery and thus reflects the adequacy of resuscitation. Blood transfusion improves the circulation and oxygen delivery, which will be further enhanced by relief of cardiac tamponade, arrest of haemorrhage, and the subsequent administration of calcium or inotropes if necessary. Haemorrhage from cardiac or vascular lacerations arrested by tamponade may rebleed fatally if such injuries are not identified before resuscitation raises the arterial and intracardiac pressures. Major injuries such as aortic transsection and cardiac disruption, as well as major airway damage and diaphragmatic rupture, can usually be diagnosed from the chest radiograph. Chest radiography and analysis of arterial blood gas tensions must be performed as part of the primary survey and within 10 minutes of the patient's admission.

Blood gas tensions, acid-base balance, and the circulatory/haemodynamic status of the patient require arterial and central venous lines for assessment of baseline values and to monitor accurately and interpret the effects of resuscitation.

Other immediately life-threatening injuries

Airway obstruction
    See chapter 3.

Tension pneumothorax
    A tension pneumothorax develops when air enters the pleural space either through the chest wall or from the lung without any means of escape. The lung on the affected side collapses completely and as the volume of air in the pleural cavity continues to increase the mediastinum and trachea are progressively shifted to the opposite side. This shift impairs venous return and then compresses the other lung further compromising ventilation.

Tension pneumothorax is a clinical diagnosis. It is recognised by respiratory distress, tracheal deviation away from the affected side, unilateral absence of breath sounds, and possibly distended neck veins. The treatment is immediate decompression; this should not be delayed by performing a chest radiograph. Insertion of a needle into the second intercostal space in the midclavicular line confirms the diagnosis and decompresses the pleural space. Following this intravenous access is obtained and an intercostal drain is placed in the pleural cavity through the fifth intercostal space anterior to the midaxillary line.

Intercostal drainage

(1) Preferentially use the fourth or fifth intercostal space between the mid- and anterior axillary lines

(2) Surgically prepare the skin, drape the chest, and infiltrate the skin and periosteum with local anaesthetic. Advance the needle above the rib to infiltrate the pleura and then confirm the presence of air or blood on aspiration

(3) Incise the skin down to the rib and then develop the track above the rib by blunt dissection. This avoids damage of the intercostal bundle

(4) Once the pleura has been punctured a gloved finger must be inserted into the pleural cavity before any drain is placed. This ensures that the incision is in the correct place and prevents damage to the lung or other organs

(5) Do not use the trocar to force the drain through the chest wall but introduce it with the tip of a large surgical artery forceps (for example, Roberts'). The drain should slide into position easily through the track already made, and be directed towards the apex of the chest cavity

(6) Attach the tube to an underwater seal drainage system

(7) When the drain is in position secure with zero gauge suture. A pursestring suture is also applied

(8) Check the position and efficacy of the drain in a chest radiograph

(9) Do not clamp the tube after insertion

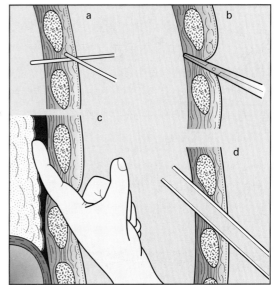

Chest drain insertion. (*a*) Penetration of the skin, muscle, and pleura. (*b*) Blunt dissection of the parietal pleura. (*c*) Exploration of the pleural cavities. (*d*) Tube directed posteriorly and superiorly.

Chest injuries

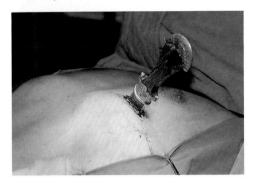

Knife wound in the chest. The knife moved with the cardiac cycle.

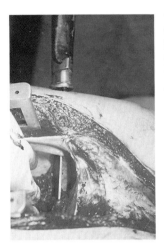

The knife transfixed the pericardium and lacerated but did not penetrate the inferior surface of the heart. The patient left hospital after four days.

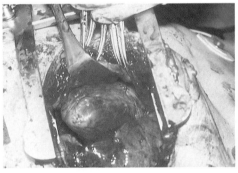

Exposure of the heart for immediate repair of a cardiac stab wound.

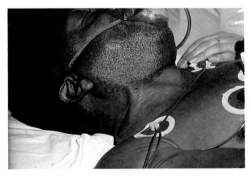

Patient with a cardiac stab wound and tamponade. The neck veins are greatly distended despite blood loss.

Open pneumothorax

Although most penetrating injuries usually seal off, larger defects may remain open, causing a sucking chest wound. There is immediate equilibration between intrathoracic and atmospheric pressures, and if the defect is large enough air will pass preferentially through the defect with each respiratory effort appreciably reducing respiratory efficiency. The defect should be covered initially with a sterile occlusive dressing secured on three sides to act as a flutter valve, and an intercostal drain must then be inserted away from the open wound. Surgical closure will be necessary later.

Massive haemothorax

Although massive haemothorax is usually caused by a penetrating injury it may also result from blunt trauma. It is defined as occurring when more than 1500 ml of blood is lost within the chest cavity or drain. The signs are those of hypovolaemic shock associated with absent breath sounds and dullness to percussion on the affected side. The neck veins may be collapsed secondary to hypovolaemia, or dilated and full because of the mechanical effects of a chest cavity full of blood or associated tension pneumothorax or cardiac tamponade. Massive haemothorax is managed by simultaneously decompressing the chest cavity and restoring the blood volume. Rapid crystalloid infusion through large calibre intravenous lines is started and changed to type-specific blood if possible or cross matched blood as soon as it is available. A large bore intercostal drain (32 French gauge or larger) can then be inserted anterior to the midaxillary line through the fifth intercostal space. Until a cardiac or vascular injury has been ruled out the systemic pressure should not be allowed to rise uncontrollably as this may precipitate further bleeding and cause death. The amount of continuing blood loss if greater than 200 ml/h dictates the need for thoracotomy. The patient should have a central line placed in addition to large bore peripheral cannulas in preparation for rapid transfusion and monitoring clinical response. Penetrating wounds medial to the nipple or scapula should raise the index of suspicion of damage to the heart, great vessels, and hilar structures.

Flail chest

Severe crush injuries often cause extensive disruption of the chest wall with multiple rib and sternal fractures. When a segment of the chest wall loses bony continuity with the thoracic cage it becomes flail and will move paradoxically on inspiration and thus reduce the tidal volume and compromise ventilation. The principle cause of hypoxia after flail chest, however, is severe underlying pulmonary contusion. Rib fractures may be accompanied by significant blood loss. Diagnosis is by observation of abnormal chest wall movement and the palpation of crepitus. The chest radiograph will not always reveal rib fractures or costochondral separation. Full lung expansion must be restored by intermittent positive pressure ventilation if required, and draining any haemopneumothorax.

The aim of further management is to preserve respiratory function. Pain reduces the tidal volume causing inadequate ventilation of the basal segments, resulting in atelectasis. Pain also inhibits coughing, allowing secretions to obstruct bronchi and cause acute respiratory failure. Effective pain relief is required for regular physiotherapy to be carried out with the patient's full cooperation. The injured lung is sensitive to inadequate perfusion subsequent to shock and also fluid overload; therefore careful management is essential. A flail segment in itself does not justify mechanical ventilation; the degree of respiratory distress and hypoxia determines this need. Functional not physical integrity is the aim. Adequate analgesia and careful fluid management are essential. Operative stabilisation of rib fractures is rarely indicated.

Cardiac tamponade

Although penetrating injuries are usually responsible for cardiac tamponade, blunt trauma may damage the heart or great vessels causing bleeding into the pericardium. Only a small amount of blood

Pericardiocentesis

(1) Attach the patient to an electrocardiograph before starting. The vital signs and central venous pressure should also be monitored

(2) Prepare the skin surgically and infiltrate the subxiphoid area with local anaesthetic

(3) Puncture the skin 1–2 cm inferior to the left xiphochondral junction with a wide bore plastic-sheathed needle (at least 15 cm in length). Initially at 45 degrees, the needle should then be aimed towards the tip of the left scapula—the base of the pericardium

(4) As the needle is advanced simultaneously aspirate until it fills easily with blood without ECG disturbance. Then aspirate as much blood as possible

(5) ECG changes such as widening/enlarging of the QRS complex or marked ST changes suggest that the needle is too far advanced and must be withdrawn. Serious damage of the heart is rare, though injury of the posterior descending branch of the right coronary artery is possible

(6) Positive pericardiocentesis must be followed by surgical exploration

within the fixed, fibrous pericardium will restrict cardiac function severely.

Beck's triad of elevated central venous pressure, hypotension, and muffled heart sounds may not be present; the neck veins in a hypovolaemic patient can be empty and the nature of the heart sounds difficult to assess in a noisy emergency room. Kussmaul's sign of paradoxical elevated venous pressure on inspiration associated with tamponade may be present.

Pericardiocentesis is indicated in patients suspected of cardiac tamponade who have failed to respond to initial resuscitative measures. The removal of as little as 20 ml of blood can improve the condition of a critically ill patient considerably. Although pericardiocentesis may be life saving in certain circumstances, it has also caused death through cardiac laceration and should therefore be performed with caution. A fine balance between the internal and external cardiac pressures prevents exsanguination in cardiac tamponade; aspiration of blood from the pericardium may cause further fatal haemorrhage by allowing a rise in intracardiac pressure and removing the tamponading effect. If the patient is moribund attempted pericardiocentesis should not be allowed to delay immediate thoracotomy.

Patients with a positive pericardiocentesis must undergo surgical exploration and inspection of the heart. If the blood within the pericardium has clotted aspiration will not be possible; this occurs in about 25% of cases.

Secondary survey

The plain chest radiograph

- This is the single most important investigation in patients with thoracic trauma
- Perform within 10 minutes of the patient's arrival
- The ideal position is erect, though this is often not possible
- Enables a good assessment of the amount of blood or free air within the chest
- Enables diagnosis of serious injuries such as, cardiac tamponade, aortic laceration, diaphragmatic laceration, and major airway disruption

Once the immediately life-threatening conditions have been diagnosed and treated or excluded the patient can be assessed thoroughly. This assessment includes a detailed history and a full examination as well as chest radiograph, measurements of arterial blood gases, and electrocardiography. Plain chest radiography is the most important investigation in patients with thoracic trauma, and should be performed with the patient erect if possible, though in practice it is often done with the seriously injured patient in a supine or partially erect position. An erect film enables the best assessment of lung expansion and free air or blood in the chest cavity. Widening and shift of the mediastinum as well as rib fractures may be evident. Serious injuries such as cardiac tamponade, transsected aorta, ruptured diaphragm, and major airway injury can usually be diagnosed from the chest radiograph. Multiple rib fractures, fractures of the first or second ribs, or scapular fractures indicate severe force being delivered to the chest and its internal organs. Pneumomediastinum or pericardium or air beneath the deep cervical fascia suggest tracheobronchial disruption. Surgical emphysema of the chest wall and haemopneumothorax are often indicative of pulmonary laceration following rib fractures.

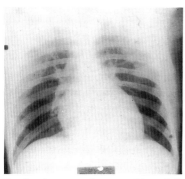

Cardiac tamponade caused by a left parasternal stab wound.

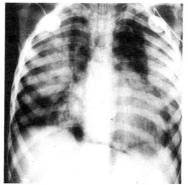

Free air in the mediastinum and beneath the deep cervical fascia owing to tracheal transection.

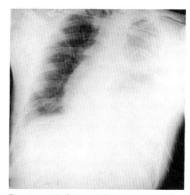

Ruptured left hemidiaphragm with haemothorax and stomach and ruptured spleen in left pleural cavity.

Potentially lethal injuries

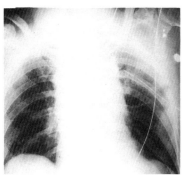

Aortic transsection caused by a deceleration accident.

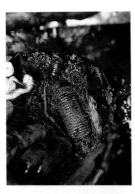

Traumatic transsection of the thoracic aorta repaired by a Dacron tube graft.

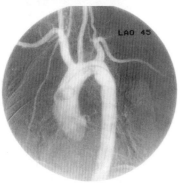

Aortogram showing laceration at the usual site after a deceleration injury.

The following injuries are often missed in the primary survey as they are not immediately life-threatening. They are, however, all very serious injuries which may cause death.

Pulmonary contusion

The insidious development of the respiratory distress syndrome following pulmonary contusion makes this injury potentially lethal. There is associated atelectasis and shunting of blood, decreased lung compliance, and increased airway resistance. The resulting increase in work is in addition to that caused by injury to the chest wall. Some patients can be managed without intubation and mechanical ventilation. Early intubation (within the first hour) must be considered when:
- There is hypoxia or worsening respiratory status
- The level of consciousness is impaired
- The patient is being transferred to another hospital
- There is pre-existing chronic pulmonary disease
- Surgery for abdominal or orthopaedic injuries is necessary
- Other systemic organ function failure such as ileus or renal failure occurs.

Myocardial contusion

Contusion of the heart is the most commonly undiagnosed fatal injury. It occurs when there is direct compression of the heart or with deceleration trauma. It is often associated with sternal fractures; in such cases the right ventricle is more commonly damaged. Chest pain is usually assumed to be due to chest wall contusion or rib fractures. The diagnosis is established from the mechanism of injury, electrocardiographic changes, serial cardiac enzyme measurements; and two dimensional echocardiographic evidence of ventricular wall dysfunction, and pericardial effusion. Sinus tachycardia, multiple ventricular ectopics, atrial fibrillation, non-specific ST and T wave changes, and conduction abnormalities such as right bundle branch block may be seen. An area of contused myocardium behaves as an area of infarction would, and the patient should be treated accordingly. The complications are those of myocardial infarction and are treated the same. Conduction defects may require a pacemaker. Cardiogenic shock is rare but some patients may need intra-aortic balloon pumping to improve the perfusion of viable myocardium. Urgent repair using cardiopulmonary bypass is necessary for cardiac rupture, ventricular septal rupture, or valve avulsion.

Ruptured aorta

Tears of the aorta or pulmonary arteries are immediately fatal in 90% of cases. They usually occur as a result of blunt injuries. The aorta may be completely or partially transsected or have a spiral tear. The commonest site of rupture is at the attachment of the ligamentum arteriosum at which point the aorta remains fixed throughout any deceleration injury. The immediate survival of the patient depends on the development of a contained haematoma, maintained by intact adventitia. The survival of patients after reaching hospital is dependent on early diagnosis followed by surgical repair.

Any suspicion of aortic injury raised by the plain chest radiograph must lead to further investigation. No single radiographic sign predicts aortic rupture, although a widened mediastinum is the most consistent finding.

Further investigation by should be undertaken in the hospital where surgery will be performed. If transfer is necessary the patient should be mechanically ventilated and the systolic blood pressure kept below 100 mm Hg using infusions of sodium nitroprusside or propanolol, or both.

The treatment of traumatic aortic rupture is surgical repair either directly or by resection of the damaged segment and interposition of a vascular graft. This should take priority over all other surgical procedures except control of life-threatening haemorrhage.

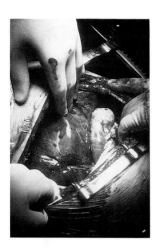

Ruptured left hemidiaphragm with the stomach in the chest.

Diaphragmatic rupture

Penetrating chest injuries cause small diaphragmatic perforations that are rarely of immediate significance. By contrast blunt trauma produces large radial tears of the diaphragm and easy herniation of abdominal viscera. The right hemidiaphragm is relatively protected by the liver and left sided ruptures are therefore more common; they are also more easily diagnosed because of the appearance of gut in the chest. Bilateral rupture is rare. The chest radiograph can be misinterpreted as showing a raised hemidiaphragm, acute gastric dilatation, or a loculated pneumothorax. Contrast radiography or locating the abnormal position of the stomach on plain radiography with a nasogastric tube confirms the diagnosis. Unless intracranial injuries or potentially fatal haemorrhage require immediate surgery then repair of the diaphragm should not be delayed. This is often performed through a laparotomy for associated abdominal injuries.

Major airway injury

Extensive free air in the neck, mediastinum, or chest wall should always raise suspicions of major airway damage. Laryngeal fractures are rare. They are indicated by hoarseness, subcutaneous emphysema, and palpable fracture crepitus. Attempted intubation is warranted if the airway is completely obstructed or there is severe respiratory distress. The airway may be hazardous to secure and require immediate tracheostomy followed by surgical repair.

Transsections of the trachea or bronchi proximal to the pleural reflection cause extensive deep cervical or mediastinal emphysema, which readily spreads to the subcutaneous tissues. Injuries distal to the pleural sheath lead to pneumothoraces. Blunt tracheal injuries may not be obvious, particularly if the conscious level is depressed. Penetrating injuries are usually apparent and require surgical repair. They can be associated with injury of adjacent structures, most commonly the oesophagus, carotid artery, or jugular vein. Missile injuries can involve extensive tissue damage to the surrounding area from the blast effect.

Laboured breathing may be the only indication that there is airway obstruction. Bronchoscopy, preferably rigid to improve airway clearance of blood and debris, confirms the diagnosis and early surgical repair is required. Injury to a major bronchus is usually the result of blunt trauma. There are often severe associated injuries and most victims die at the site of the accident; for those who reach hospital there is a 30% mortality. Signs of bronchial injury may include haemoptysis, subcutaneous emphysema, tension pneumothorax, and pneumothorax with a large persisting air leak. Most bronchial injuries occur within 2·5 cm of the carina and the diagnosis is confirmed by bronchoscopy. Mucosal oedema and debris can obscure the extent of a bronchial injury so the site should be carefully inspected. Distortion of airway anatomy by adjacent haematoma makes management more difficult, and surgery is occasionally indicated. Bronchial tears must be repaired early through a thoracotomy.

Indications for thoracotomy after initial resuscitation

- Cardiac tamponade
- Massive air leak suggestive of major airway injury
- Initial chest drainage >1500 ml, or three consecutive hours of >200 ml/h blood loss
- Chest wall defects
- Diaphragmatic lacerations

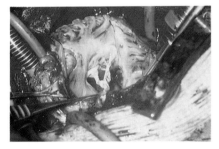

Lacerated tricuspid valve after a blunt cardiac injury. The valve was repaired on cardiopulmonary bypass.

Oesophageal trauma

Damage to the oesophagus is usually caused by penetrating injury. Blunt oesophageal injury is rare. It occurs after a severe blow to the upper abdomen. Gastric contents are forced up into the oesophagus producing a linear tear through which they are then able to leak. Mediastinitis and rupture into the pleural space with empyema formation follow. The clinical picture may be identical to that of spontaneous rupture of the oesophagus. Although the diagnosis is often delayed, it is not difficult to make once the possibility of rupture is considered.

The diagnosis is confirmed by contrast study of the oesophagus or endoscopy. Treatment is by surgical repair and drainage of the pleural space through a thoracotomy.

Signs of oesophageal injury

- Left pneumothorax or hydrothorax without rib fractures
- Mediastinal air
- Gastric contents in the chest drainage
- Pain or shock out of all proportion to the apparent injury

---

5 HYPOVOLAEMIC SHOCK

Peter J F Baskett

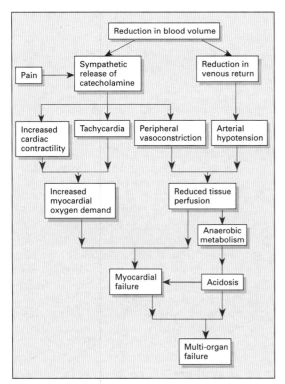

Hypovolaemic shock is a clinical state in which tissue perfusion is rendered relatively inadequate by loss of blood or plasma after injury to the vascular tree.

A reduction in blood volume produces a fall in systolic pressure, which triggers a sympathetic catecholamine response that results in peripheral vasoconstriction, a rise in pulse rate, and a reduction in pulse pressure. The tachycardia and increased cardiac contractility lead to an increased myocardial oxygen requirement.

Blood flow to the skin and peripheral tissues is reduced in an effort to preserve reasonable perfusion of vital organs such as the brain, heart, liver, and kidneys. If there is continuing blood loss inadequate tissue perfusion results in anaerobic metabolism, acidosis, and reduction in the performance of the vital organs. Further myocardial depression accelerates this process, and pain stimuli add to the sympathetic outburst.

The following are early symptoms and signs of hypovolaemic shock. They reflect the underlying pathophysiology.

- Tachycardia (due to catecholamine release)
- Skin pallor (vasoconstriction due to catecholamine release)
- Hypotension (due to hypovolaemia, perhaps followed by myocardial insufficiency)
- Confusion, aggression, drowsiness, and coma (due to cerebral hypoxia and acidosis)
- Tachypnoea (due to hypoxia and acidosis)
- General weakness (due to hypoxia and acidosis)
- Thirst (due to hypovolaemia)
- Reduced urine output (due to reduced perfusion)

In most cases the signs and symptoms can be related to the amount of blood loss, which can be classified in four broad groups (classes I–IV).

Classification of hypovolaemic shock according to blood loss (adult)

	Class I	Class II	Class III	Class IV
Blood loss:				
Percentage	<15	15–30	30–40	>40
Volume (ml)	750	800–1500	1500–2000	>2000
Blood pressure:				
Systolic	Unchanged	Normal	Reduced	Very low
Diastolic	Unchanged	Raised	Reduced	Very low or unrecordable
Pulse (beats/min)	Slight tachycardia	100–120	120 (Thready)	>120 (Very thready)
Capillary refill	Normal	Slow (>2 s)	Slow (>2 s)	Undetectable
Respiratory rate	Normal	Tachypnoea	Tachypnoea (>20/min)	Tachypnoea (>20/min)
Urinary flow rate (ml/h)	>30	20–30	10–20	0–10
Extremities	Colour normal	Pale	Pale	Pale, clammy, and cold
Complexion	Normal	Pale	Pale	Ashen
Mental state	Alert	Anxious or aggressive	Anxious, aggressive, or drowsy	Drowsy, confused, or unconscious

Symptoms of hypovolaemia according to blood loss

Blood loss (ml)	Class	Symptoms
<750	I	None
– 1500	II	Cardiovascular signs due to catecholamine release: thirst, weakness, tachypnoea
– 2000	III	Systolic pressure falls
>2000	IV	Systolic pressure becomes unreadable

Generally, losses of up to 750 ml (class I) (15% of the circulating blood volume) do not generate any pronounced signs or symptoms. Further haemorrhage, amounting to 1.5 litres (class II), produces cardiovascular signs of catecholamine release, thirst, weakness, and tachypnoea. Systolic pressure begins to fall as blood loss mounts to 2 litres (class III) and often becomes unrecordable after 2.5–3.0 litres (class IV) have been lost.

In previously healthy young adults systolic pressure is often preserved despite quite appreciable blood loss (1.5–2.0 litres) owing to the effective response to sympathetic stimulation. A narrowed pulse pressure is often the earliest sign. Eventually, however, there is a precipitous fall as the myocardium suddenly fails because of hypoxia and acidosis. Conversely, patients with coronary arterial disease may become hypotensive because of myocardial insufficiency after only modest blood losses of up to 500 ml.

Patients receiving certain drugs (for example, β blockers) may not be able to produce an appropriate sympathetic response and may also become hypotensive after modest blood loss. Other factors that may modify the response to blood loss include the patient's age, the extent of tissue damage, and the period of time between injury and examination.

In children normal haemodynamic values are maintained until the loss is relatively great. Tachycardia and skin pallor are the earliest signs, and hypotension indicates uncompensated shock with severe blood loss and inadequate resuscitation. As a rule a child's systolic blood pressure is 80 mm Hg plus twice the age in years. The diastolic is about two thirds of the systolic pressure. A systolic pressure of 70 mm Hg or less in a child therefore indicates serious cardiovascular decompensation.

In elderly patients, however, hypotension may be an early sign of blood loss. Their physiological reserves are reduced and they are less able to respond to release of catecholamines by tachycardia. The ensuing hypotension may result in early organ failure because of hypoperfusion, and this is exaggerated in normally hypertensive patients.

Extensive tissue damage from major limb injuries is associated with early cardiovascular decompensation, not only because of blood loss and haematoma formation but also because of extravasation of fluid while oedema is developing. About a quarter of the volume of oedema fluid is contributed by lost plasma volume, and this may amount to 20%–30% of the overt blood loss. Clearly oedema formation increases with time and this becomes more important as the time between injury and examination increases.

The objective of the management of hypovolaemic shock is to maintain tissue oxygenation and restore it to normal values. This entails applying the basic principles of resuscitation of patients with trauma. Resuscitation is followed by definitive treatment (including surgery).

Resuscitation of patients with trauma

(1) Adequate pulmonary oxygenation

(2) Control of haemorrhage

(3) Replacement of lost volume

(4) Monitoring the effects of (1), (2), and (3)

(5) Support of myocardial contractility

(6) Relief of pain

Pulmonary oxygenation

Ventilate patients with hypovolaemic shock
Use 100% oxygen for patients with severe shock

To ensure optimal pulmonary oxygenation patients with hypovolaemic shock should have a clear airway and be adequately ventilated with oxygen at a high inspired concentration. Unconscious patients with severe shock should be intubated and ventilated with 100% oxygen, and care should be taken to exclude impairment of ventilation due to pneumothorax, haemothorax, or diaphragmatic elevation caused by gastric distention.

Control of haemorrhage

For peripheral haemorrhage:
"Parts in the air, press on the hole"

Peripheral haemorrhage should be controlled by elevation of the injured part and by placing a firm pad and bandage over the wound ensuring adequate pressure. Tourniquets are rarely advised though may be essential and are relatively harmless in patients who are going to undergo amputation. Probing the wound to search for ruptured vessels is not recommended.

Replacement of loss

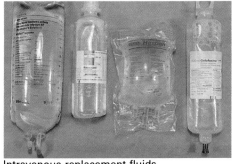

Intravenous replacement fluids.

Blood loss should be replaced intravenously in response to clinical signs and symptoms and in all patients estimated to have lost more than 750 ml.

Intravenous cannulation

The site of haemorrhage should be considered carefully when cannulation is undertaken. There is little point in setting up an infusion in an injured limb or in the femoral vein in a patient with pelvic or abdominal injuries. With this proviso the peripheral veins of the arm, if accessible, are traditionally preferred for cannulation.

The diameter of the cannula in a cannula over needle system should

Hypovolaemic shock

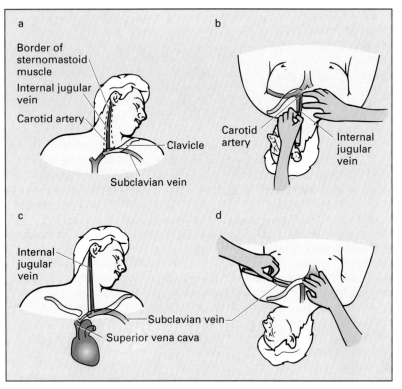

a
Border of sternomastoid muscle
Internal jugular vein
Carotid artery
Clavicle
Subclavian vein

b
Carotid artery
Internal jugular vein

c
Internal jugular vein
Subclavian vein
Superior vena cava

d

Cannulation of the jugular vein ((a) and (b)) and of the subclavian vein ((c) and (d)). Remember that the neck should not be turned until cervical spine injury has been excluded both radiologically and clinically.

Intravenous fluid replacement in haemorrhagic shock

Class I (haemorrhage 750 ml (15%))	2.5 l Ringer-lactate solution or 1.0 l polygelatin
Class II (haemorrhage 750 − 1500 ml (15–30%))	1.0 l polygelatin plus 1.5 l Ringer-lactate solution
Class III (haemorrhage 1500–2000 ml (30–40%))	1.0 l Ringer-lactate solution plus 0.5 l polygelatin plus 1.0–1.5 l whole blood or 1.0–1.5 l equal volumes of concentrated red cells and polygelatin
Class IV (haemorrhage >2000 ml (40%))	1.0 l Ringer-lactate solution plus 1.0 l polygelatin plus 2.0 l whole blood or 2.0 l equal volumes concentrated red cells and polygelatin or hetastarch

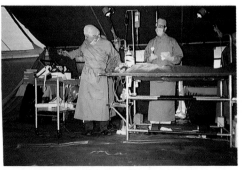

Intravenous infusion in military surgery.

be not less than 14 gauge.

Peripheral venous access may, however, be technically difficult in a shocked patient with a shut down circulation. The other options are a surgical cut down technique or percutaneous access to a central vein by the Seldinger method. The method selected will depend largely on the physician's skill and experience.

A surgical venous cutdown may be done on the long saphenous vein at the site of the medial malleolus or the saphenous vein in the groin. Access in the groin permits the introduction of a wide bore cannula or even a giving set or nasogastric tubing for rapid infusion. If access to the saphenous vein is difficult or contraindicated, the brachial or cephalic veins in the antecubital fossa are suitable. A surgical cut down is relatively time consuming except in expert hands, but it does provide reliable venous access.

Percutaneous central venous access may be achieved through the internal jugular, subclavian, or femoral veins, and the choice will depend on the possibility of damage to the cervical spine and the site of injury, as well as the expertise and experience of the operator. These central veins are less liable to constrict during blood loss and may be engorged by tilting the patient head down for the internal jugular and subclavian routes and head up for the femoral. The Seldinger technique is usually preferable, and permits insertion of a 10 gauge short cannula for rapid infusion. Long lines inserted from the antecubital fossa are not usually suitable for rapid infusions as the flow rate is inversely proportional to the length of the catheter.

Central venous access can be achieved rapidly but success rates are related to practice and expertise. The method can be unreliable, and even experts fail sometimes.

Choice of intravenous fluid

Warmed intravenous fluids should be given to restore an adequate circulating blood volume. Normal electrolyte and coagulation constituents, colloid osmotic pressure, and a packed cell volume above 30% are necessary to ensure adequate oxygen carrying capacity. The choice of intravenous fluids in clinical practice lies among crystalloid, colloid, and albumin solutions; blood in the form of whole blood or packed red cells; and a judicious mix of all of these. An example is shown in the box.

In the United Kingdom departments vary as to the fluids they use and whether they transfuse blood. It is important to realise, however, that colloid solutions replace intravascular loss and restore haemodynamic values towards normal, but they do not replace interstitial loss. In contrast, crystalloid solutions replace both interstitial and intravascular loss, but large volumes are required to restore normal haemodynamics.

Crystalloid solutions—Ringer's lactate solution may be used in patients with mild class I haemorrhage of up to 15% of blood volume. Replacement volumes should be three to four times the estimated loss as the electrolyte solution is distributed throughout the extracellular (intravascular and interstitial) space. The volume should be increased to compensate for urine loss. Vascular support with isotonic electrolyte solutions is short lived.

Colloid solutions are generally iso-oncotic and may be used to replace lost volumes of blood on a 1:1 basis, restoring haemodynamic variables to normal values. Polygelatins are cheap and effective blood volume expanders. They have a long shelf life of six years, a half life in vivo of six to eight hours, and a low index of causing anaphylactic reactions. Haemaccel has a similar electrolyte content to plasma whereas Gelofusine contains very little potassium. Both are suitable for replacing blood losses of up to 1 litre and in patients with more extensive haemorrhage when used in combination with blood transfusion to maintain a packed cell volume of 30%.

Hetastarch (6% in isotonic saline) is an effective blood substitute in patients with mild and moderate blood loss. It is more expensive than the polygelatins but has a much longer half life (12 to 14 hours) in the circulation. Care must be taken, therefore, to avoid circulation overload when blood is transfused at a later stage to restore the packed cell volume. The incidence of anaphylactic reactions is low.

Blood—Whole blood or packed red cells are required in patients with moderate and major blood loss to maintain a packed cell volume of 30%. It is not desirable to strive for higher values in the early stages of volume resuscitation as a modest reduction in packed cell volume allows improvement in the microcirculation, especially in the presence of arteriolar vasoconstriction.

Though whole blood is the ideal replacement in patients with major haemorrhage, limitations of supply may dictate that concentrated red cells are used, diluted to normal values of packed cell volumes by concurrent transfusion of polygelatin or hetastarch.

Trauma and obstetric centres should retain a small number of relatively fresh units of O negative blood for immediate transfusion in cases of severe, life threatening haemorrhage.

Blood transfused rapidly should be warmed before infusion to maximise flow rates and to minimise the risk of cardiac arrhythmia and core hypothermia. Blood filters have not been proved to be of value.

Autologous blood—In patients with severe thoracic or abdominal injuries "clean" blood may be aspirated from the cavity, anticoagulated, and returned to the patient through an intravenous cannula using a "cell saver" system. Autologous blood is valuable in patients with major vascular injuries of the thorax and abdomen and in those with a ruptured liver or spleen. Clearly, however, the procedure cannot be applied in patients with abdominal trauma who have a ruptured bowel or in those with thoracic trauma who have oesophageal or lung damage. The transfusion of autologous blood has several advantages, particularly if the patient's blood group is uncommon. The blood is the patient's own, free of infection, warm, and immediately available.

Coagulation problems

Coagulation problems occur in patients with massive blood loss because of dilution with blood substitutes and the fact that coagulation factors deteriorate rapidly in stored blood. Moreover, tissue destruction releases various products that inhibit the normal coagulation process. The clotting process should be monitored by regular screening and deficiencies treated definitively rather than by infusion of valuable fresh frozen plasma and platelets on an arbitrary basis.

Disadvantages of blood transfusion in hypovolaemic shock

- Time is required to group and cross match individual units of blood
- Blood has a high viscosity and the microcirculation in shock may be improved by a reduction in packed cell volume
- Blood stored for more than a few days has a high potassium ion concentration and the platelets and white cells fragment rapidly, losing normal function
- Blood and certain blood products may be infected. (The risk of acquiring HIV infection from transfused blood has been virtually eliminated in the United Kingdom)

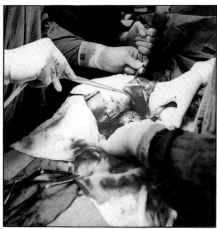

Aspiration of "clean" blood from the cavity.

Monitoring progress and treatment

Variables to monitor

- Respiration rate
- Pulse rate
- Arterial pressure
- Pulse pressure
- Central venous pressure
- Urinary output
- Changes in the electrocardiogram
- Temperature
- Peripheral oxygen saturation
- End tidal carbon dioxide levels
- Mental state

Requirements for blood volume replacement should be based on all of the factors in the box, particularly pulse rate, arterial pulse and central venous pressures, peripheral oxygen saturation, and urine flow rates. Transfusion should be continued to produce an adequate arterial pressure, a urine flow of 50 ml/h, and a central venous pressure that responds to a rapid infusion of 200 ml by a sustained rise of more than 3 cm H_2O over the previous value.

If these variables improve and the improvement is maintained then clearly the blood loss is under control. Failure to maintain the improved values indicates continuing loss and requires further transfusion and early surgery. If the patient does not respond satisfactorily to transfusions the rate of loss is exceeding the fastest possible rate of intravenous replacement. This is usually associated with major thoracic, abdominal, or pelvic injuries. In such instances the

Hypovolaemic shock

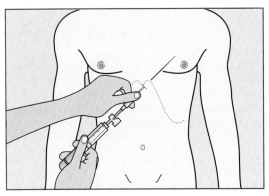

Needle pericardiocentesis.

patient must be taken to the operating room for immediate thoracotomy, laparotomy or external fixation of the pelvis with the bleeding controlled by clamps, packs, or both. In this way the anaesthetist can "catch up" with the transfusion requirements. Salvage of autologous blood may be appropriate.

A rising central venous pressure associated with a low arterial pressure, tachycardia, and a reduced urine output indicates tension pneumothorax, cardiac tamponade, or cardiac failure. Cardiac tamponade is treated by thoracotomy, sometimes preceded by relief needle paracentesis. In patients requiring inotropic support because of myocardial failure measurement of pulmonary wedge pressure and cardiac output with a pulmonary artery flotation catheter or a Doppler ultrasound probe may be helpful in comparing individual ventricular load and performance. In most patients with previously normal hearts, however, the central venous pressure and the pulmonary artery wedge pressure follow each other closely and the extra expense of this invasive technique is unjustified.

Maintenance of normal carbon dioxide and oxygen tensions will optimise cerebral perfusion.

Cardiac contractility and renal output

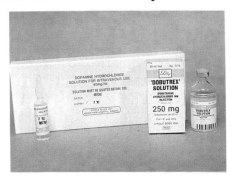

Inotropic drugs.

A patient with a previously impaired myocardium may need inotropic support with dopamine and dobutamine. Such support is not a substitute for adequate volume replacement but is used to enhance myocardial contraction if required. Rates of dopamine infusion should be confined to "renal" doses (up to 5 µg/kg/h) that enhance urine output. Higher doses cause vasoconstriction and tachycardia, which results in an increase in myocardial oxygen demand that may not be achievable because of inadequate myocardial blood flow. Dobutamine should then be added to improve myocardial performance.

Pain relief

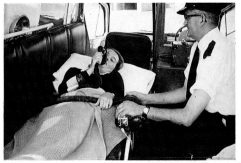

Patient receiving Entonox on the way to hospital.

Pain relief must be given not only for its compassionate value but also for its essential beneficial influence on the pathophysiology of hypovolaemic shock in reducing catecholamine secretion. Giving a mixture of 50% nitrous oxide and 50% oxygen (Entonox) is of value before the patient reaches hospital, and this should be supplemented with increments of intravenous morphine 5 mg, nalbuphine 10 mg, or ketamine 25–50 mg with diazepam 5–10 mg or midazolam 5 mg until analgesia is achieved. Metoclopramide 10 mg should also be given intravenously if an opiate is given.

Conclusion

The photograph showing aspiration of blood was reproduced by kind permission of Solco Basle and that of needle pericardiocentesis by Mosby Europe.

Many patients will die of hypovolaemic shock despite the fact that the principles of management and treatment are well known and understood. Too often, however, in retrospect the treatment offered was too little, too late, allowing a malignant circle of pathophysiological changes to be irreversibly established. Early aggressive treatment offers the best results.

Pneumatic anti-shock garment

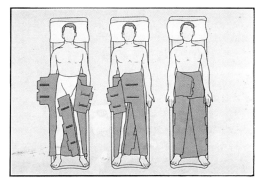

Pneumatic counter pressure suit.

Pneumatic antishock garments (medical antishock trousers) have been used extensively, particularly in the United States, to control haemorrhage from the legs, pelvis, and abdomen and spinal shock. The suit consists of inflatable sections for each leg and the abdomen and is radiotranslucent with access for urinary catheterisation and digital rectal examination.

Application of the suit produces:

- Autotransfusion of 0.5–1.5 litres of homologous blood
- Reduction in haemorrhage from tissues beneath the suit
- Reduction in the total functioning volume of the vascular compartment, permitting relatively improved perfusion of the heart, brain, and arms (thereby assisting with intravenous cannulation)
- Splinting of limb and pelvic fractures with consequent reduction in blood loss and pain.

- Do not apply the abdominal section in pregnant women or patients with abdominal injury with protruding viscera
- Do not deflate the suit until at least two wide bore intravenous cannulas are safely in situ and an adequate supply of blood and blood substitute are available
- In patients with abdominal injuries or ruptured aortic aneurysm the suit should not be deflated until the patient is in the operating room and the surgical team ready to control haemorrhage
- Do not leave the suit inflated for more than two hours as ischaemic anaerobic metabolism may lead to profound general metabolic acidosis
- Take care not to overtransfuse patients with poor left ventricular function with the suit inflated because pulmonary oedema may occur
- The suit is contraindicated in cases of left ventricular failure, ruptured diaphragm, or pulmonary oedema.

The suit should be applied in patients with symptoms of hypovolaemia and a systolic blood pressure <90 mm Hg. Suit inflation pressures of 40–50 mm Hg (5.5–6.5 kPa) should be used initially, increasing to 80 mm Hg (10.5 kPa) if the systolic pressure does not improve. The time of application should be noted.

Pneumatic counter pressure suits are being used less often in the United Kingdom, and even in the United States where their acceptability is a matter of strong debate. It is likely that the time spent in putting them on would be better used in ensuring rapid transfer to hospital, particularly in urban areas where the distance between accident site and hospital is short. The suit may be useful if the travelling time exceeds 45 minutes.

6 HEAD INJURIES

Ross Bullock, Graham Teasdale

Staff in an accident and emergency department serving a population of 250 000 people can expect to treat about 5000 patients each year who have suffered a head injury—10% of their work. Most attenders are only mildly injured, but head injuries have a reputation for being treacherous. A traumatic intracranial haematoma will develop in fewer than 12 patients each year but can transform an initially mild injury into a life threatening emergency. In the small number of patients (less than 5%) who present with persistent impaired consciousness correct diagnosis and assignment of priorities can be life saving. The limited availability of specialist neurosurgical facilities in the United Kingdom means that doctors can admit only 1% of the patients who attend with head injuries to a neurosurgical unit.

Role of accident and emergency and trauma staff in management of head injuries

- Resuscitate, diagnose, and record
- Detect or exclude other injuries
- Request, supervise, and interpret results of radiography and other initial investigations
- Decide if admission is needed and if so, where
- Liaise with other specialties—for example, neurosurgery—about serious cases
- Ensure adequate arrangements for observing and maintaining patient's condition during transfer to other departments or hospitals
- Observe progress of patients with minor injuries, who should be admitted to short stay beds
- Ensure adequate arrangements for follow up

In recent years the task for staff in accident and emergency departments has been simplified by the development of agreed guidelines for management, thus reflecting the increased knowledge of the mechanisms of head injury, improved methods of assessment and diagnosis, and more accurate identification of patients at risk of brain damage.

The two main aims of management of patients with head injuries are, firstly, to provide the best conditions for recovery from any brain damage already sustained and, secondly, to prevent or treat complications leading to secondary brain damage.

Mechanisms of brain damage

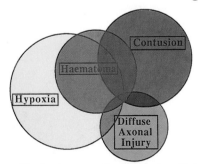

Causes of brain damage after severe head injury.

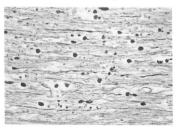

Retraction balls—the microscopic feature of diffuse axonal injury.

Diffuse damage
The brain is poorly anchored within the skull and its soft consistency renders it liable to move within the skull in response to acceleration or deceleration.

Contact between the surface of the brain and the interior skull causes bruising (contusions), particularly at the frontal and temporal poles. Distortion of the brain caused by internal shearing forces leads to stretching and tearing of axonal tracts within the white matter. Such diffuse axonal injury manifests itself as microscopic retraction balls at the site of damaged fibres; these are widespread in severe injuries, but mild stretch injury with reversible loss of function is also responsible for the transient disturbance of consciousness known as "concussion".

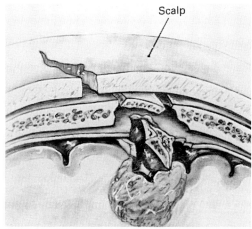

Compound depressed skull fracture.

Focal impact damage

Skull fracture—At the point of impact the skull deforms inwards and fracture may occur. Such fractures are less common in children than in adults because of their more elastic skulls.

A compound depressed fracture results when a violent sharp blow cavity, sometimes tearing the dura mater. Should the brain surface be exposed then this is known as an open fracture. This injury is an important source of intracranial infection and requires prompt surgical elevation and debridement. A depressed fracture is also a powerful cause of epilepsy, but the risk of this complication is not influenced by surgical treatment.

A linear fracture is important chiefly as an indicator of potential secondary intracranial bleeding.

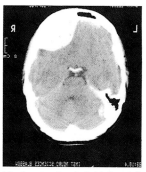

Moderate sized right frontal extradural haematoma.

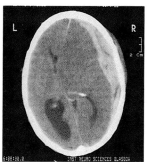

Large right subdural haematoma with pronounced midline shift and contralateral ventricular dilatation.

Extradural haematoma—The inbending of the skull may strip off underlying dura and create a space in which an extradural haematoma develops. This can be associated with little primary brain damage, and optimal management should minimise mortality and morbidity due to secondary cerebral compression. Delayed treatment can cause irreversible cerebral damage.

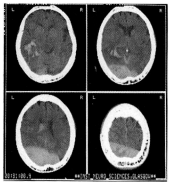

Large occipital extradural haematoma overlying confluence of intracranial venous sinuses with left temporal contusion.

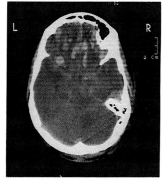

Multiple bifrontal cerebral contusion caused by a fall on to the occiput (a "contra-coup" injury).

Intradural haematoma—Subdural and intracerebral bleeding are four times more common than extradural haematoma. They result from tearing of cerebral veins or from laceration of the brain's surface, or both. An association with primary brain damage is common, but the outcome may nevertheless be good if an operation is performed promptly.

Hypoxia and ischaemia

The brain requires continuous perfusion with well oxygenated blood. Permanent ischaemic neuronal damage occurs if this is reduced below a critical threshold for more than a few minutes. Normally the brain regulates its own blood supply to maintain constant perfusion despite wide variations in systemic blood pressure; when injured, the brain loses this capacity and is thus particularly vulnerable to ischaemic damage when hypotension or hypoxia occur.

A reduction in mean arterial blood pressure to below 60–80 mm Hg, particularly when intracranial pressure is raised, may cause ischaemic neuronal damage if sustained for more than a few minutes. Multiply injured patients may become severely shocked immediately after injury.

When a head injury is severe enough to produce unconsciousness early respiratory disorders and bradycardia occur and are a potent cause of ischaemic damage. The airway is often compromised immediately after injury owing to mechanical obstruction or loss of protective reflexes.

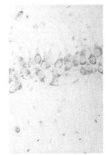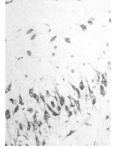

Normal hippocampal neurones (left); shrunken, pyknotic hippocampal neurones irreversibly damaged by ischaemia or hypoxia (right).

Head injuries

Causes of raised intracranial pressure after head injury

- Haematoma
- Focal cerebral oedema related to a contusion or haematoma
- Diffuse oedema after ischaemia (cytotoxic)
- Diffuse brain swelling ("brain engorgement")
- Obstruction of cerebrospinal fluid pathway (this is rare)

Raised intracranial pressure

About 70% of patients persistently in coma after severe head injury have raised intracranial pressure. This jeopardises cerebral perfusion because cerebral perfusion pressure is equal to mean arterial blood pressure minus intracranial pressure.

As intracranial pressure rises cerebrospinal fluid is driven out of the intracranial compartment—the first stage in compensation. As the pressure continues to rise brain shifts occur within the cranial cavity.

The most important of these brain shifts is uncal transtentorial herniation or "coning". This causes impairment of conscious level, development of a fixed dilated pupil, and brain stem compression with cardiovascular and respiratory abnormalities.

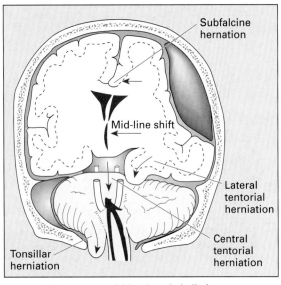

Intracranial contents within closed skull show shifts in response to haematoma.

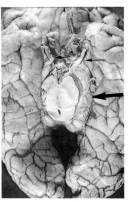

Midbrain sectioned at level of third cranial nerves shows uncal transtentorial herniation or "coning" (large arrow). Note bilateral "notching" of third nerves due to compression against tentorium (small arrows).

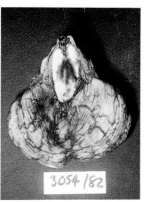

Consequences of unrelieved brainstem compression: "flame shaped" brainstem haemorrhage with irreversible damage to vital centres.

Management of head injuries

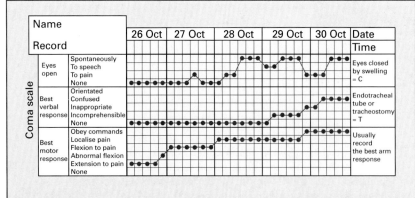

For patients with a depressed conscious level the first priority is to stabilise circulation and respiration and prevent further secondary cerebral damage. The risks of secondary complications then need to be assessed and a decision made regarding transfer to a neurosurgical centre.

Additional factors

In addition to the factors recorded on the Glasgow coma chart the following should be recorded:

- Pupil diameter and reaction to light
- Pulse and blood pressure
- Temperature and respiration
- Movement of all limbs

All patients require ongoing recording of conscious level (by the Glasgow coma scale)—the best motor response should be used. To exclude traumatic tetraplegia the response to painful stimuli should be tested by supraorbital nerve compression if limb responses are absent. Patients observed may be either in hospital or, in certain cases, at home, provided that the patient can be discharged into the care of a responsible adult.

Management of patients who cannot talk

- *Airway with cervical spine control*—Definitive control of airway; immobilise cervical spine
- *Breathing*—Analysis of blood gas tensions (Po_2 >13 kPa (100 mm Hg) and Pco_2 <5.3 kPa (40 mm Hg) is acceptable)
- *Circulation*—Restore haemodynamic stability
- *Dysfunction of central nervous system*—Check score on coma scale, pupils, limb movements
- *Exposure and radiographs*—Remove all clothing and examine "head to toe" (as described in chapter 1). Obtain skull, chest, and cervical spine radiographs rapidly and ensure that the top of the T_1 vertebra is imaged. If there is doubt obtain a computed tomogram of the cervical spine

Priorities for management depend on whether the patient can talk. If he or she cannot do so both intracranial and extracranial complications are more likely.

In patients who can talk, document their history, duration of amnesia after trauma, mechanism of injury, previous medical and surgical history, and previous intake of drugs and alcohol.

In all cases after the secondary survey has been completed give prophylactic antibiotics for leakage of cerebrospinal fluid, basal skull fracture, compound fracture, or depressed fracture—for example, give penicillin two million units intravenously six hourly for seven days or orally as appropriate or co-trimoxazole 960 mg twice daily for seven days orally.

Indications for endotracheal intubation in patients with severe head injuries

- Absent gag reflex when oropharyngeal suction is attempted in unconscious patients
- When airway protection is needed—for example, when there is oropharyngeal bleeding, facial fracture, or vomitus that cannot be easily cleared by the patient
- When ventilation or blood gas tensions, or both, are too poor to allow spontaneous ventilation. (PaO_2 <9 kPa breathing air or <13 kPa when receiving supplemental oxygen; $Paco_2$ >5.3 kPa.) (Exclude pneumothorax on the basis of the chest radiograph)
- To allow hyperventilation when a patient's condition is deteriorating because of raised intracranial pressure (discuss with a neurosurgeon)

Guidelines for endotracheal intubation

If injury of the cervical spine has not been excluded intubate the patient with the neck stabilised by an assistant or by using sandbags. A full stomach should always be assumed and a rapid sequence of induction employed, with cricoid compression. Not all intubated patients require artificial ventilation.

Short acting drugs (for example, thiopentone, etomidate, propofol, and suxamethonium, atracurium, and vecuronium) should be used to facilitate intubation, which should be performed by an experienced person (usually an anaesthetist).

A cuffed endotracheal tube should be used, except in young children, and securely fixed to the patient with a neck halter and adhesive strapping. After intubation adjust the position of the tube to ensure that air entry is present in both lungs as intubation of the right main bronchus is common. An anaesthetist (or other experienced person) should accompany an intubated patient during transfer within the hospital or between hospitals.

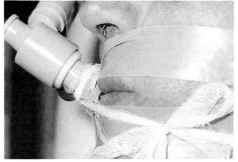

Intubated patient with head injury. Note secure fixation of endotracheal tube.

Indicators for skull radiography

If any of the following are present skull radiography should be performed:
- Neurological symptoms and signs
- Cerebrospinal fluid or blood from the nose or ear
- Suspected penetrating injury (it may be necessary to shave the hair)
- Pronounced bruising or swelling of the scalp.

Hospital admission

Example of a head injury warning card

(Accident and emergency department tel   )

This person has recently sustained a head injury and should be kept under regular observation every two hours for the first 24 hours. The person should be asked to tell you his or her name, where he or she is, the year, and who you are and should show you that he or she can move all four limbs normally. If asleep you should awaken the person to do these tests. If the person develops any of the following problems he or she should be brought back to hospital without delay:

(1) Drowsiness or excessive sleepiness

(2) Confusion or disorientation

(3) Severe headaches, vomiting, or fever

(4) Weakness of any limbs or double vision

(5) Convulsion, seizure, or passing out

(6) Discharge of blood or fluid from ears or nose

The following list of indications for admission of patients with head injuries should be displayed in accident and emergency departments.

- Confusion or any other depression of consciousness at the time of the examination
- Skull fracture
- Neurological symptoms or signs, or both
- Difficulty in assessing the patient—for example, because of ingestion of alcohol, epilepsy, or other medical conditions that cloud consciousness; children are also difficult to assess
- Lack of a responsible adult to supervise the patient and other social problems.

Brief amnesia after trauma with full recovery is not necessarily an indication for admission.

If the patient is to be observed outside hospital he or she should be discharged with a head injury "warning card" into the care of a responsible person.

The aims of hospital admission are to provide optimal conditions for recovery of the brain and to detect complications before they cause further secondary brain damage. The mainstay of admission is therefore neurological observation, which should be hourly for at least the first 24 hours.

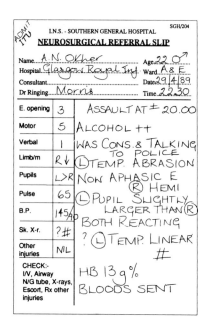

Consultation with a neurosurgeon

A group of British neurosurgeons formulated the following list of indications for consultation with a neurosurgeon and computed tomography in patients with head injuries.

(1) Fractured skull with confusion or worse impairment of consciousness, focal neurological signs, fits, or any other neurological symptoms or signs.
(2) Coma continuing after resuscitation, even if there is no skull fracture (coma is defined as not obeying commands, not speaking, not opening eyes—that is, a Glasgow coma score <8).
(3) Deterioration in level of consciousness or development of other neurological signs.
(4) Confusion or other neurological disturbance persisting for more than six to eight hours with or without skull fracture.
(5) Compound or open depressed fractures of the vault of the skull.
(6) Suspected fracture of the base of the skull—causing leakage of cerebrospinal fluid, orbital haematoma, or mastoid haematoma—or other penetrating injury (for example, gunshot wounds).

Patients in categories 1–3 should be referred and scanned urgently. In all cases the diagnosis and initial treatment of serious extracranial injury takes priority over transfer to the nearest neurosurgical unit to avoid hypotension during both the transfer and the neurosurgical management.

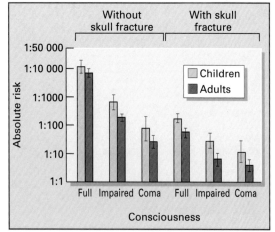

Absolute risk of intracranial haematoma in patients with head injury.

Computed tomography

Increasing numbers of accident and emergency departments have access to emergency computed tomography for patients with head injuries, but the interpretation of the computed tomogram is often difficult—for example, features of raised intracranial pressure can be missed by the untrained observer. It is preferable for computed tomography to be performed under the control of a neurosurgeon or neuroradiologist.

Drugs in acute head injury

Antibiotics in head injury

Indications

Basal fracture
Open vault fracture
Suspected or proven meningitis

Suitable agents

Benzylpenicillin 1 million units intravenously every six hours for seven days or phenoxymethylpenicillin orally 500 mg every six hours (children 10–20 mg/kg/day)

For patients with penicillin allergy give oral co-trimoxazole 960 mg twice daily

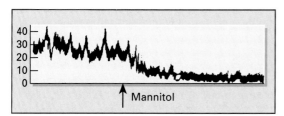

The effect of mannitol in a patient with raised intracranial pressure after severe focal brain injury.

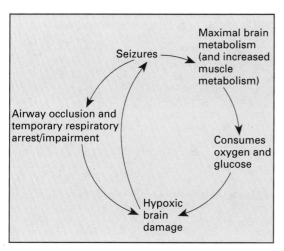

The consequences of uncontrolled seizures.

Sedation and analgesia

Sedation and analgesia for patients with head injuries are often a problem; they may be in pain and nauseous as a result of their injury, yet strong opiate analgesics and drugs with respiratory depressant effects must be avoided as they may cause iatrogenic deterioration in conscious level and respiratory depression. For adults give paracetamol 250–500 mg every six hours or dihydrocodeine preparations such as DF118, or Cocodamol one to two tablets every four to six hours. If given parenterally DF118, 30 mg every six hours is usually safe and effective. Give metoclopramide 10 mg up to every eight hours for nausea intravenously or orally. For children paracetamol suspension 125–250 mg every six hours is suitable.

Antibiotics

The choice of antibiotic for an established infection—for example, hypostatic pneumonia, wound, or intracranial infection—should be guided by identification of the causative organism and its sensitivity. Prophylactic antibiotics should be avoided, and their value is controversial because of the risk of developing resistant infection. It is essential to seek advice from the local neurosurgeon.

Mannitol

Mannitol is a powerful osmotic diuretic and may be life saving, but it carries dangers. It should be used, in consultation with a neurosurgeon, to "buy time" while the patient is prepared for transfer to the nearest neurosurgical centre. Give 0.5–1 g/kg as a bolus over 10–30 minutes. (Usually 250–400 ml of a 20% solution for adults.)

Steroids

Several trials have shown no benefit from steroids, even at high doses.

Management of seizures

Seizures within the first week carry a low risk of future epilepsy but may cause severe hypoxic brain damage. Prevent further seizures with phenytoin as a loading dose of a 10–15 mg/kg bolus given intravenously over 20 minutes (with electrocardiography) followed by an intravenous infusion of 250–500 mg over four hours. Thereafter give 100 mg every eight hours intravenously or orally.

If seizures persist after phenytoin loading give clonazepam 0.25 mg intravenously incrementally after each seizure. Be prepared to ventilate the patient in an intensive care unit. Intravenous diazepam 5–10 mg may be used if seizures still persist but may cause respiratory depression.

Restlessness

In patients with head injury restlessness is often a warning sign, and restless patients should not be sedated without excluding hypoxia, hypotension, metabolic derangement, a full bladder, or pain due to other injuries. The "checklist" for secondary deterioration described below should be considered before sedation is prescribed.

Secondary deterioration in conscious level

Effect of hypotension and hypoxia on patients' outcome after acute head injury

	Outcome	
	Dead/ vegetative/ severely disabled	Moderate disability, good recovery
Both hypoxia and hypotension	6	
Hypoxia only	11	7
Hypotension only	1	1
Neither hypoxia nor hypotension	11	38

$\chi^2 = 14.72$; $p<0.005$.

If deterioration in conscious level is apparent the following possibilities should be investigated.

Hypoxia—Check arterial blood gas tensions, respiratory rate, and chest radiographs. Start or continue treatment with oxygen.

Ischaemia—Check pulse, blood pressure, electrocardiogram, and full blood count, particularly if there has been a substantial delay between the patient sustaining the head injury and assessment. Exclude intra-abdominal bleeding (consider peritoneal lavage).

Head injuries

Metabolic derangement—Exclude dehydration and check urea, electrolyte, and blood glucose concentrations.

Missed intracranial haematoma—If hypoxia, ischaemia, and metabolic derangement have been excluded repeat computed tomography urgently.

Seizures—Seizures may not have been witnessed. Control them with drugs. Consult a neurosurgeon.

Meningitis—If meningitis is suspected first obtain a computed tomogram to exclude the presence of a haematoma, which may cause neck stiffness. Start treatment with high doses of antibiotics immediately. Lumbar puncture should be performed only after computed tomography has excluded raised intracranial pressure. (Appropriate antibiotic treatment is intravenous penicillin 5 million units every six hours and intravenous chloramphenicol 1–2 g every six hours.)

Exploratory burr holes

The use of exploratory burr holes in modern management of head injury is extremely limited. Even experienced neurosurgeons miss one third of intracranial haematomas and may initiate bleeding and worsen brain damage. Use of burr holes may be indicated if a capable surgeon is available and a previously alert patient rapidly deteriorates and develops a fixed dilated pupil that is ipsilateral to a skull fracture and in patients whose transfer to a neurological centre is likely to take two hours or more.

Interhospital transfer

The events associated with interhospital transfer are a potent cause of avoidable mortality and morbidity after head injury. Problems are caused by:

- Delay in arranging transfer
- Inadequate resuscitation before transfer
- Inadequate preparation for the journey
- Inadequate care during the ambulance journey.

Patients with hypovolaemia who have not been fully resuscitated may become profoundly hypotensive during an ambulance journey. Patients in a coma should be intubated before transfer and accompanied by a doctor who has the experience and equipment necessary to cope with any eventuality.

Outcome after severe head injury

Outcome at six months after head injury related
to age, best coma score, and best pupil reaction
at 24 hours after injury

	Dead or vegetative (%)	Moderate disability or good recovery (%)
Age:		
0–29	39	50
30–59	49	34
≥60	81	11
Coma score:		
3–5	84	11
6–7	56	29
8–10	28	58
11–15	16	72
Pupils:		
Both fixed	86	6
One or both reacting	16	72

Moderate and severe deficits in patients with
head injuries. Figures are percentages of patients

	Degree of overall disability	
	Moderate	Severe
Physical handicap		22
Cognitive impairment	8	78
Personality change	18	89

The main determinants of outcome are coma scale score at admission, age, pupillary state, raised intracranial pressure, and the presence of hypoxia or ischaemia. About 40% of patients who are in a coma after initial resuscitation and beyond six hours after injury will die. Prognosis should not be estimated too soon because resuscitation and stabilisation may dramatically improve the patient's conscious level.

Late sequelae

Neurological recovery after severe injuries takes about two years but is most rapid within the first six months. Mental disabilities are far more important for the patient and his or her family than physical impairment. Personality changes, poor motivation, impaired memory and concentration, and lack of emotional restraint are the most common of these. They often cause difficulty with schooling, employment, and family relationships, and patients should be advised against returning to school or employment too soon after a head injury. Psychometric testing often discloses unsuspected difficulties and allows more directed rehabilitation to be formulated.

Common physical sequelae include ataxia, hemiparesis, speech disorders, cranial nerve palsies such as anosmia, unilateral blindness, diplopia, unilateral deafness, and tinnitus. Seizures occur in 4% to 40% of patients, depending on the nature of the initial injury, focal injuries being more epileptogenic.

Symptoms after minor head injury

Proportion (%) of patients with certain
neurological symptoms after trauma

	At discharge	At one year
Headache	36	18
Dizziness	17	14
Depression	8	18

The illustration of a skull fracture was reproduced from Rob and Smith's *Operative Surgery: Neurology* by kind permission of the publishers, Butterworth, and that of intracranial contents from *Neurology and Neurosurgery Illustrated* by kind permission of the publishers, Churchill Livingstone.

In a third of patients with minor head injury symptoms such as headache, dizziness, irritability, poor concentration, tinnitus, poor balance, fatigue, depression, and intolerance of alcohol will persist for more than six months. Many of these "postconcussional" symptoms are due to mild diffuse axonal injury, and occur in patients who have been unconscious for only a few minutes and who may have electrophysiological and neuropsychological abnormalities. The symptoms usually subside spontaneously; depression and anxiety may lead to their persistence but malingering is rare. When the symptoms begin only after an appreciable interval psychological factors are likely to be more important.

Specific treatment for postconcussional symptoms is lacking. In the early stages reassurance that severe brain damage has not occurred is important, but patients should not resume activity too rapidly. If the patient has difficulty in coping, anxiety and depression may be provoked and lead to perpetuation of symptoms. Psychotherapeutic support is appropriate, but the value of more formal psychological rehabilitation is not proved. Analgesics are appropriate in the early stages, but the smaller their effect the greater the need for a psychological approach.

7 MAXILLOFACIAL INJURIES

Iain Hutchison, Michael Lawlor, David Skinner

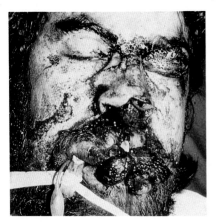

Management of the airway

The multiply injured patient may have injuries of the face and neck that are life threatening or sufficiently serious to require specialist advice and management. In the initial assessment such patients may present with airway obstruction or hypovolaemic shock due to profuse and continuous bleeding from the facial skeleton or its surrounding soft tissues. The resuscitation team must be aware of these problems, know which specialists to call and when to call them, and be able to initiate manoeuvres to prevent the demise of the patient before the arrival of the specialist.

The first priority of the resuscitation team is to secure and maintain an airway, yet this action transgresses the site of maxillofacial trauma, which may be littered with broken teeth and dentures, bits of fractured bone, and macerated soft tissue.

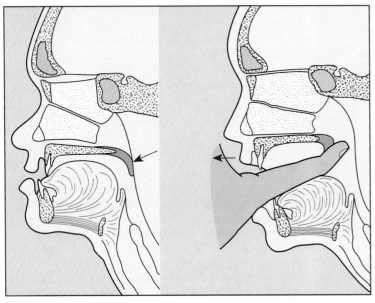

(Left) Fractured maxilla with posterior displacement, causing obstruction of the nasopharynx (arrowed). (Right) Fractured maxilla disimpacted and pulled forward to clear airway.

Six specific problems associated with maxillofacial trauma may affect the airway:

(1) A fractured maxilla may be displaced posteroinferiorally along the inclined plane of the base of the skull, blocking the nasal airway.

Management—Disimpact by pulling the maxilla forward with the index and middle fingers in the mouth behind and above the soft palate and with the thumb on the region of the incisors.

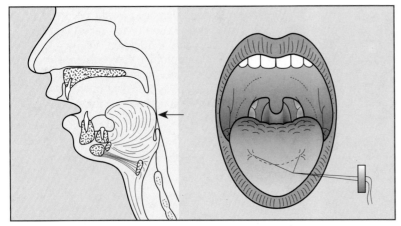

(Left) Fractured mandible with loss of anterior attachment of the tongue. The tongue drops back, blocking the airway (arrowed). (Right) Traction suture in the tongue taped to the face.

(2) The tongue may lose its anterior insertion in patients with a bilateral anterior mandibular or symphyseal fracture. It may then drop back in a supine patient, blocking the oropharynx.

Management—Insert a deep traction suture (0 gauge black silk) transversely through the dorsum of the tongue and tape the suture on to the side of the face; or, if no suture is available, pull the tongue forward by using a towel clip or pull the mandible forward manually.

36

Indications for chest radiography or bronchoscopy, or both

- A foreign body is unaccounted for
- Cyanosis, tachypnoea, tachycardia, and respiratory distress
- Deterioration in PaO_2

(3) Teeth, dentures, bone fragments, vomitus, haematoma, and other foreign bodies may block the airway at any site from the oral cavity through the oropharynx, larynx, and trachea down to the bronchi, especially the right main bronchus.

Management—(a) Clear the oral cavity by using a gloved finger inserted laterally (just inside the cheek) to the back of the mouth, then hook the finger medially and forward to pull debris out of the mouth. (If the finger is pushed centrally foreign bodies may be pushed further down the airway.) (b) Repeat this manoeuvre from the opposite side of the mouth. (c) Use a large bore sucker (plastic yankauer) and good illumination to aspirate the oral cavity. (d) Use the laryngoscope and sucker (ignoring potential pain from mandibular fractures) to examine and clean the oropharynx and larynx.

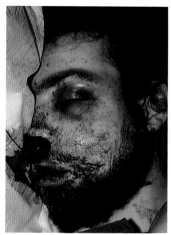

Life threatening haemorrhage from a closed bony injury of the maxilla.

(4) Haemorrhage may result from several causes:
(i) Distinct vessels in open wounds.

Management—Insert 5 cm ribbon gauze or gauze swabs as a firm compressed pack into the open wound to achieve pressure, request cross matching of blood, and arrange for definitive treatment.

(ii) The nose, as a result of damage to the anterior or posterior ethmoidal vessels or the terminal portion of the maxillary artery (see management of bleeding).

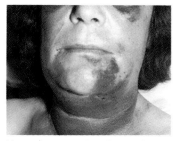

Haematoma and oedema of the neck and floor of the mouth caused by a fractured mandible.

After dealing with these immediate problems consider orotracheal intubation.

(5) Soft tissue swelling and oedema. Trauma of the oral cavity causes swelling around the upper airway. This rarely presents an immediate problem, but the swelling may worsen insidiously over a few hours and cause later airway problems.

Management of injuries of the larynx and trachea that threaten the airway

- If the injury is above the larynx
  —Perform cricothyroidotomy
- If the injury is at the level of the larynx and is incomplete
  —Experts may pass an endotracheal tube
  —Otherwise, seek specialist opinion for tracheostomy
- If the injury is at the level of the larynx and is complete
  —Seek specialist opinion for tracheostomy
- If the injury is in the trachea, below the potential tracheostomy site
  —Refer urgently to a thoracic surgeon

(6) Maxillofacial trauma may occasionally be associated with trauma to the larynx and trachea, which may cause obstruction of the airway by swelling or displacement of structures such as the epiglottis, arytenoid cartilages, and vocal cords.

Management—(a) Maintain a high index of suspicion if the mechanism of injury suggests trauma to the larynx and trachea: for example, in cases of blunt trauma of the neck caused by impact with a steering wheel. (b) Note any neck swelling, dyspnoea, voice alteration, and frothy haemorrhage. (c) Palpate the neck for surgical emphysema (crackling), tenderness, and, before swelling progresses, laryngeal or tracheal crepitus at the site of the fracture. (d) Arrange for lateral and anteroposterior radiographs of the soft tissues of the neck and mediastinum to be taken urgently to find out whether there is air in the soft tissue. (e) If suspicion is maintained perform bronchoscopy to determine the site of injury.

Management of bleeding

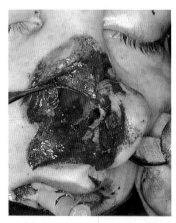

Apparently simple nasal soft tissue injury, which on exploration required extensive repair.

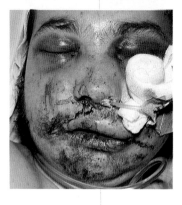

Major haemorrhage caused by closed maxillofacial trauma, treated by anterior and posterior nasal packing.

Procedure for anterior and posterior nasal packing

(1) Insert 12/14 G Foley catheters with 20 ml balloons into the nose

(2) Inflate balloons when the tip of the catheter is in the postnasal space

(3) Pull back the catheter until the balloon occludes against the choana at the back of the nose

(4) Tape the catheters under tension to the side of the face

(5) Insert bismuth iodoform paraffin paste 5 cm ribbon gauze packs into the nose in front of the balloon and Foley catheter

---

Soft tissues

Although the scalp, face, and neck have an excellent blood supply, extensive superficial lacerations in this region are not always accompanied by blood loss of such quantity that a transfusion is required. Conversely, small puncture wounds to the skin that scarcely seem to need suturing may cause life threatening haemorrhage if they involve a moderate size artery such as the facial artery or superficial temporal artery. The danger lies in overlooking the continuous trickle of fresh blood from the puncture wound.

Management—These wounds should be dealt with by senior specialist surgeons. Initial management comprises application of direct pressure to control haemorrhage. Definitive management comprises: (a) Assess wounds regularly for blood loss. (b) If haemorrhage continues explore the wounds and clip or ligate bleeding vessels. (c) Extend puncture wounds along natural skin crease lines to locate bleeding vessels. (d) If profuse bleeding occurs from a neck wound, consider whether there is enough time for arteriography, check arm pulses, extend the wound to expose the major vessels in the neck (usually along the anterior border of the sternomastoid), control the bleeding, and assess damage. Small vessels off the external carotid artery may be ligated. Large arteries (for example, the carotid and subclavian arteries) usually require repair. It is possible to ligate one internal jugular vein without untoward effect, and it may be possible to ligate one common carotid artery without causing a stroke.

Bone

Significant haemorrhage also occurs occasionally in patients with closed injuries to the bony structures of the middle third of the face—that is, the maxilla, nose, and ethmoids. This presents as a steady flow of blood from the nose and oral cavity and bleeding into the soft tissues of the face, producing profound cheek swelling with a shiny, tense skin.

Two problems exist:
 (i) Failure to recognise the extent of blood loss and subsequent development of a coagulopathy.
(ii) An inability to define the source of the arterial bleeding as fractures of the middle third of the face are usually bilateral with disruption of the nasal septum. Therefore, haemorrhage from one side manifests equally at both nostrils.

Management—(a) Exclude the possibility of bleeding from the base of skull by palpating the pharyngeal wall with your index finger through the mouth for tears and fractures. (b) Insert anterior and posterior nasal packs.

Secondary survey

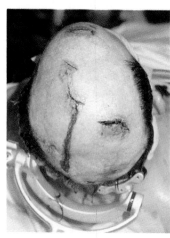

Underneath this apparently minor scalp injury was a fractured skull.

Once the airway has been secured and haemorrhage arrested the definitive management of soft tissue and bone trauma of the face and neck may be deferred until life threatening neurosurgical, thoracic, abdominal, and neurovascular limb injuries have been dealt with. It may be appropriate, however, to perform simultaneous procedures or even combined operations, particularly when cranial trauma is combined with facial trauma.

Examination

(1) Expose the affected area by cleaning all wounds and the face and scalp with Savlon (0.15% cetrimide). **Do not discard any loose bone or soft tissue fragments.**

(2) Examine the scalp for lacerations and bruises, not forgetting the back of the scalp if it is possible to move the patient—that is, if a cervical spinal injury has been excluded or the cervical spine is immobilised.

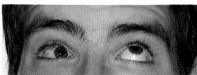

Limitation of upward gaze denoting an orbital floor fracture.

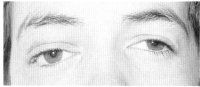

Proptosis and depression of right pupillary level due to fractured orbital roof and intraorbital haematoma.

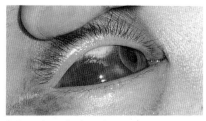

Subconjunctival ecchymosis.

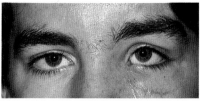

Left medial canthal damage with characteristic almond shaped palpebral fissure and increased intercanthal distance.

Indications of bleeding from the ears

Site	Indication
Anterior wall of the external auditory meatus	Fracture of the condylar neck of the mandible
Posterior wall or middle ear	Fracture of the base of the skull in the middle cranial fossa
Ecchymosis behind the ear (Battle's sign)	Probable middle cranial fossa fracture

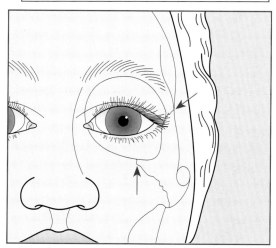

Palpate frontozygomatic and zygomaticomaxillary sutures for pain and separation.

(3) Examine the eyes for:
- Visual acuity—can the patient count fingers? Can he or she read print?
- Limitation of eye movements, diplopia, and unequal pupillary levels. If one or more of these is present suspect trauma of the orbital floor and wall with entrapment of periorbital tissues.
- Direct, consensual, and accommodation reflexes. Examination of these may help detect a rise in intracranial pressure, but be aware of false positive signs caused by trauma to the globe, resulting in post-traumatic mydriasis, and retrobulbar haemorrhage.
- Proptosis (or exophthalmos). This suggests haemorrhage within the orbital walls.
- Enophthalmos. This suggests fracture of an orbital wall (usually the floor or medial wall).
- Periorbital swelling. If this is present suspect a fracture of the zygoma or maxilla.
- Subconjunctival ecchymosis. If this is present suspect direct trauma to the globe or a fractured zygoma.

Examine the anterior chamber and fundus for evidence of direct trauma and raised intracranial pressure.

(4) Examine the nose for:
- Deformity, pain, mobility, and difficulty in breathing.
- Bleeding and leakage of cerebrospinal fluid. If present suspect anterior cranial fossa fracture at the cribriform plate. Do not pass a nasal endotracheal tube or nasogastric tube. Give prophylactic sulphonamides or chloramphenicol to prevent meningitis.
Measure the intercanthal distance. If it is >3.5 cm suspect nasoethmoidal fracture.

(5) Examine the ears for bleeding and leakage of cerebrospinal fluid.

(6) Examine the soft tissues for:
- Sensory (V nerve) (for example, of the upper or lower lip) and motor (VII nerve) deficit—this may have a peripheral or central cause. Consider this in relation to other injuries.
- Surgical emphysema around the eyes and on the face. This suggests continuity between sinuses and face due to facial fracture. To avoid emphysema instruct patients not to blow their nose. (Surgical emphysema in the face should be distinguished from that in the neck, which is caused by trauma to the larynx, trachea, or lungs.)
- Venous engorgement of the face. If present suspect trauma of the major vessels in the thorax or neck.
- Pooling of tears and leakage from the eye. This may indicate damage to the lacrimal apparatus.
- Leakage of pink or clear fluid from a facial wound. If present suspect damage to the parotid duct.

(7) Examine the face for lengthening, bilateral swelling, "panda eyes," and dish face deformity.
If any of these are present suspect bilateral maxillary fracture.

(8) Palpate around the orbit for step defects, particularly at the frontozygomatic and zygomaticomaxillary sutures. Such defects indicate fracture to the zygoma or maxilla.

(9) Palpate the mandible externally from the condyle and along the lower border for tenderness, step defects, and crepitus.

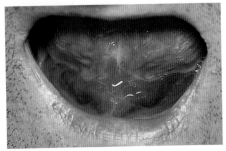

Sublingual haematoma caused by mandibular fracture.

(10) Examine intraorally for haematoma (especially under the tongue—this indicates mandibular fracture), lacerations, bleeding, loose teeth, broken teeth and dentures, mobile jaw segments, abnormal alignment of the jaw and step defects, and teeth meeting prematurely.

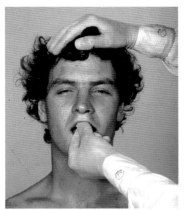

Pull on the anterior maxilla while supporting the frontal bone to show movement of the maxilla on the base of the skull, indicating maxillary fracture.

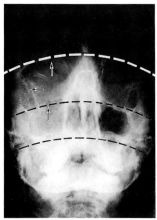

Anteroposterior occipitomental radiograph taken in the initial assessment period of a multiply injured patient. Examine along these standard arcs for evidence of fractures (arrowed).

(11) Using both hands palpate the middle third of the face for mobility. Place the thumb and fingers of the right hand on either side of the premaxillary teeth (with the thumb in front and the index finger on the palatal side). Place the palmar surface of the left hand across the forehead. Pull the premaxillary segment forward gently and see whether nose or cheek bones move, indicating a maxillary fracture at the Le Fort I, II, or III level.

(12) Good quality maxillofacial radiographs help in the definitive planning of treatment. The radiologist will decide which views are appropriate.

Conclusion

The photographs of general facial trauma and limitation of eye movements were provided by Mr D R James, those of haemorrhage by Mr J Attenborough, that of proptosis by Mr R Haskell, and that of oedema by Mr R Juniper.

Major maxillofacial injuries may occur in isolation or in combination with other injuries. They pose problems because they are intimidating and obstruct access to the airway. Rarely, they may be the cause of life threatening haemorrhage, which is often overlooked.

The definitive management of soft tissue and bone injuries of the face and neck can usually be deferred while life threatening thoracic, abdominal, and neurological injuries are dealt with. It may be appropriate, though, for the maxillofacial surgeon to help the anaesthetist and perform a fuller assessment, wound toilet, and preparatory procedures while the patient is anaesthetised. Combined procedures with specialists such as neurosurgeons may also be indicated.

8 SPINE AND SPINAL CORD

Andrew Swain, John Dove, Harry Baker

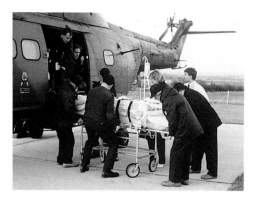

Incidence (percentage) of neurological injury in patients with fractures or dislocations of various parts of the spine

Part of spine	Incidence
Any	14
Cervical spine	40
Thoracic spine	10
Thoracolumbar junction	35
Lumbar spine	3

A patient with serious multiple injuries is rarely able to provide a coherent history. Injuries that carry a risk of death or severe disability must, therefore, be suspected from the outset so that correct early management can be instituted. Any patient with trauma who is not fully conscious should be assumed to have an injury of the cervical spine until proved otherwise. The thoracolumbar spine must also be managed carefully. The commonest reason for failing to detect an important spinal injury is failure to suspect one, particularly in patients with multiple trauma; but sometimes a serious injury is considered minor.

The spinal cord is most often damaged in the cervical region, but it is also particularly at risk near the thoracolumbar junction. The thoracic spine is splinted by ribs and sternum, but the spinal canal is narrower in this region relative to the width of the spinal cord so when vertebral displacement occurs it is more likely to damage the cord. Partial cord injuries are generally more common, and the potential for neurological improvement or deterioration is correspondingly greater.

Management at the scene of the accident

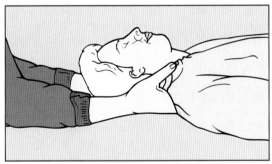

Manual immobilisation of the neck.

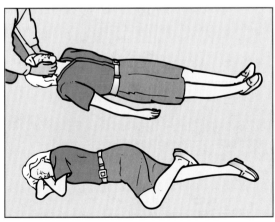

Supine position with airway protection (top); lateral recovery position (bottom).

Spinal trauma may be suspected from a witness's description of an accident. It cannot, however, be excluded without a definitive examination, even in the fully conscious patient. The neck must be aligned in the neutral position without longitudinal compression or distraction. This will improve the airway and reduce spinal deformity, helping to relieve pressure on the spinal cord or arteries. If the patient is a motorcyclist the doctor should support the neck while an assistant carefully eases the helmet off. The neck is then splinted with a rigid collar of appropriate size to grip the chin. Collars alone are inadequate and they need to be supplemented by manual stabilisation or lateral support with sandbags and forehead tape. Be wary of swelling under the collar, which may develop from a haematoma or surgical emphysema.

In the unconscious patient the airway should be opened by chin or jaw lift and an oropharyngeal airway inserted. The supine position facilitates clinical examination, cardiopulmonary resuscitation (if required), respiratory movements, and control of the neck, but tracheal intubation is required to prevent aspiration. Alternatively the patient can be turned into the lateral position with the trunk straight but inclined forwards by 20 degrees, allowing secretions to discharge freely from the mouth. The three quarters prone or coma position cannot be recommended as it entails rotation of the cervical spine and splints the diaphragm, causing hypoventilation.

Spine and spinal cord

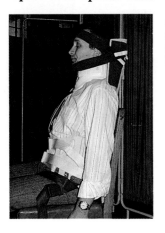

Semirigid collar and spine immobiliser.

Thoracolumbar injury must also be assumed and treated by carefully straightening the trunk and correcting rotation. The patient may be log rolled or lifted as necessary (ideally by four assistants), but it is vital that the whole spine is maintained in the neutral position.

The neck and back can be protected simultaneously in patients who are erect or supine by means of a spinal board incorporating a head immobiliser or one of the spine immobilisers, for example, Kendrick or Russell extrication devices which are lighter and can be applied to a sitting patient. Doctors should familiarise themselves with the splints that are available locally.

Transfer to hospital

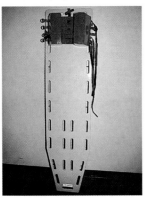

Spinal board with head immobiliser

Once the airway is protected and oxygen has been administered and the patient positioned, one or more intravenous infusions are established. If conditions allow, the patient should be examined briefly before transportation. A "scoop" stretcher can be assembled underneath a patient who is lying free and used to transfer him or her to a spinal board or ambulance stretcher. Patients in immobilisers must be carried in and not by the splint. In the absence of life threatening injury the patient with spinal trauma should be transported carefully to hospital. Hard objects should be removed from anaesthetic parts of the body.

Arrival at hospital: primary survey

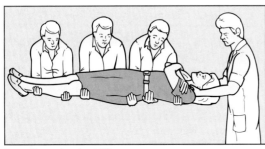

Coordinated spinal lift.

Safe transfer of the patient from the ambulance to a trauma trolley is best achieved with the patient strapped to a spinal board, which is not removed until spinal injury has been excluded. Alternatively a scoop stretcher may be used. Transfer from an ambulance stretcher in the resuscitation room can also be accomplished by four people, the person in charge grasping the base of the neck and supporting the head with his or her wrists. In this way there should be no seesaw movement of the neck if the actions of those lifting the patient become uncoordinated. Once the patient is lifted the trauma trolley can be wheeled underneath. Resuscitation is then continued while the spine is protected.

Airway (with protection of the cervical spine)

Patients with multiple trauma are invariably kept supine during resuscitation unless regurgitation occurs and the airway is unprotected. In such an emergency the patient may be tipped head down and oropharyngeal suction applied. In patients with cervical cord injury pharyngeal stimulation by vigorous suction manipulation of a Guedel airway or intubation may result in unopposed vagal discharge and cardiac arrest. This can be prevented by prior administration of atropine. Many seriously injured patients require intubation, and this is not contraindicated in patients with an unstable cervical injury. The procedure should, however, be performed whenever possible by an experienced anaesthetist and spinal movement minimised by an assistant controlling the head and limiting movement. Alternative methods of intubation that do not require the neck to be moved—for example, blind tracheal intubation and use of a fibreoptic laryngoscope—should be employed only by those with the necessary experience. Ileus develops after spinal cord injury, and a nasogastric tube is required.

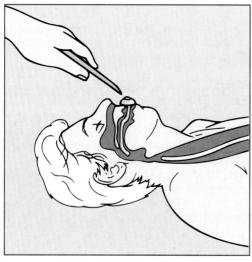

Suction: beware of vagal reflex stimulation.

Circulation

Patients with injury to the cervical cord or high thoracic cord may have reduced sympathetic outflow between the T1 and L2 segments with associated bradycardia and hypotension. Patients must be connected to a cardiac monitor on admission. Tetraplegic patients with bradycardia should be given atropine if their pulse rate drops below 50 beats/min. Haemorrhage is the commonest cause of post-traumatic shock but bradycardia with hypotension is not a classical feature of hypovolaemic shock, and in a traumatised patient it should increase suspicion of spinal cord injury. The extent of bradycardia and hypotension in neurogenic shock depends on the level and extent of neurological injury. If the systolic blood pressure falls below 80 mm Hg inotropic support is necessary. Bradycardic shock is also seen in elderly patients and patients taking β blockers.

In recent years the importance of maintaining adequate tissue perfusion and oxygenation in patients with spinal cord trauma has been emphasised. Episodes of hypotension or hypoxia often lead to irreversible neurological deterioration. Patients with spinal trauma are likely to have hypovolaemia owing to other injuries. Circulatory volume must be restored, but aggressive fluid replacement is detrimental in patients with purely neurogenic hypotension as it precipitates pulmonary oedema. Therefore traumatised patients with bradycardia and hypotension should be subjected to a fluid challenge and the response observed and monitored by measuring central venous pressure. For this, cannulation of the subclavian vein is recommended as access to the internal jugular vein is difficult to obtain without rotating the neck.

Treat

- Bradycardia—pulse rate <50 beats/min
- Hypotension—systolic blood pressure <80 mm Hg
- Inadequate urinary excretion

Do not rotate the patient's neck during central venous cannulation unless cervical injury has been excluded by both radiographic and clinical assessment

---

Secondary survey

Any injury to the spinal cord carries a high risk of early and late medical complications. Important early complications include respiratory failure due to intercostal paralysis or partial phrenic nerve palsy, impaired ability to expectorate, and ventilation-perfusion mismatch. The patient's respiratory state may also deteriorate shortly after admission as a result of ascending oedema in the traumatised cervical cord. Care must be taken in giving narcotic analgesics as these will further impair respiration. Cardiac arrest usually results from respiratory failure. Blood gas tensions and vital capacity must be checked. Pulse oximetry is important.

Abdominal trauma is not easily assessed in tetraplegic patients as the abdominal wall is anaesthetic, flaccid, and areflexic and ileus results from the neurological injury. A useful positive sign is pain at the tip of the shoulder that is aggravated by abdominal palpation. Peritoneal lavage is a particularly useful diagnostic aid in patients with cervical or thoracic cord injury.

Acute retention will develop in paraplegic and tetraplegic patients unless the sacral segments are spared. Measurement of urine output in patients with multiple trauma is important, and the bladder will usually require drainage, particularly if the patient has been drinking. In the absence of urethral trauma a narrow gauge Silastic catheter with a small (5 ml) balloon is passed under strictly aseptic conditions and taped to the anterior abdominal wall to prevent unnecessary movement of and injury to the urethra, which may lead to sepsis. Alternatively a suprapubic catheter can be inserted.

The conscious patient

Sensory loss or motor symptoms should never be disregarded, no matter how unimportant they seem. Diagnosis of spinal cord injury relies on symptoms and signs of pain in the spine with sensory loss and disturbances in motor function distal to a neurological level. The pain may radiate owing to nerve root irritation. A full neurological examination must be performed, including testing of cranial nerves, sensation to fine touch and pin prick, proprioception, power, tone, coordination, and reflexes.

Causes of respiratory insufficiency

In tetraplegic patients
- Intercostal paralysis
- Partial phrenic nerve palsy—immediate —delayed
- Impaired ability to expectorate
- Ventilation-perfusion mismatch

In paraplegic patients
- Variable intercostal paralysis according to level of injury
- Associated chest injuries—rib fractures, pulmonary contusion, haemopneumothorax

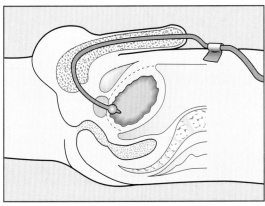

Method of catheterisation in patients with spinal cord injury.

Spine and spinal cord

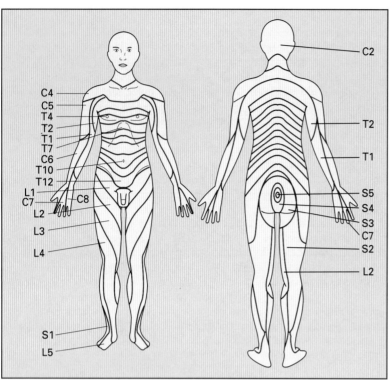

Myotomes		Reflexes	
Muscle group		*Nerve supply*	
Diaphragm		C(3),4,(5)	
Shoulder abductors		C5	
Elbow flexors		C5,6	Biceps jerk C5,6
Supinators/pronators		C6	Supinator jerk C6
Wrist extensors		C6	
Wrist flexors		C7	
Elbow extensors		C7	Triceps jerk C7
Finger extensors		C7	
Finger flexors		C8	
Intrinsic hand muscles		T1	Abdominal reflex T8-12
Hip flexors		L1,2	
Hip adductors		L2,3	
Knee extensors		L3,4	Knee jerk L3,4
Ankle dorsiflexors		L4,5	
Toe extensors		L5	
Knee flexors		L4,5 S1	
Ankle plantar flexors		S1,2	Ankle jerk S1,2
Toe flexors		S1,2	
Anal sphincter		S2,3,4	Bulbocavernosus reflex S3,4
			Anal reflex S5
			Plantar reflex

Sensory and motor neurological assessment.

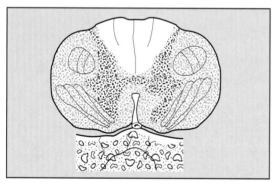

The central cord syndrome.

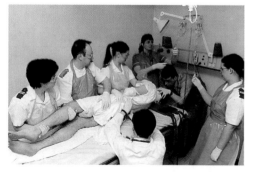

The anterior cord syndrome.

Great care must be taken in managing conscious patients as the neurological symptoms and signs may be dismissed if they do not fit a classical pattern. In patients with a partial cord lesion some neurological function is preserved distal to the level of injury (for example, the sacral segments may be spared): a vascular lesion may be responsible for this. Sometimes the zone of cord injury lies centrally, encroaching on the cervical segments of the long tracts and producing flaccid weakness in the arms (the central cord syndrome). Anterior contusion affects the spinothalamic and corticospinal tracts and is therefore associated with weakness and impaired pain and temperature sensation (the anterior cord syndrome). Posterior cord injury causes loss of sense of vibration and proprioception (the posterior cord syndrome). Trauma may be confined to one side of the cord, produces ipsilateral weakness and impaired contralateral pain and temperature sensation (Brown-Séquard "hemisection"). The central cord syndrome is more common in elderly patients in whom the spinal canal has been narrowed by cervical spondylosis. Patients with this syndrome may not have an associated fracture or dislocation, whereas those with anterior cord injury usually do. Brown-Séquard lesions are more common in patients with penetrating trauma and blunt rotational injury.

The unconscious patient

There are no truly pathognomonic features of spinal cord injury, but important signs are flaccid paralysis, diaphragmatic breathing, priapism, hypotension with bradycardia, and upward movement of the umbilicus on tensing the abdomen—this is due to a T10 lesion (Beevor's sign). Examination of the *whole* length of the spine *must* be performed in all unconscious patients with multiple trauma. Failure to do so has resulted in diagnoses being missed, with serious consequences.

The patient is log rolled to one side, keeping the spine in the neutral position. If performed correctly this is quite safe. Inspection may detect bruising, swelling or a kyphos; palpation may allow tenderness, an increased interspinous gap, or malalignment of spinous processes (rotational deformity) to be detected. Suspicion of an injury to the upper cervical spine may be aroused by a retropharyngeal haematoma seen through the open mouth; the trachea may be deviated.

Log roll.

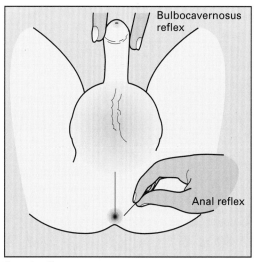

Sacral reflexes.

Neurological examination is mandatory in all unconscious patients, and baseline observations are extremely important in patients with spinal injury, not least for medicolegal reasons. Use of a Glasgow or similar coma chart will allow limb movements and strength to be charted. Some head injury charts do not include this facility. Neurological examination in unconscious patients is usually limited to completing the coma chart, funduscopy, and assessing tone and reflexes, but in patients with suspected cord injury the abdominal, anal, and bulbocavernosus reflexes should be recorded. The sensory response to pain can also be assessed in patients with depressed consciousness. Beware of flaccidity and areflexia in an arm as this may result from brachial plexus injury or spinal cord trauma, or both (particularly in motorcyclists).

Radiology

Good quality radiographs are essential for accurate diagnosis of spinal injury, and these are best obtained in the radiology department if circumstances allow. When spinal injuries are suspected radiographic examination should be supervised by a doctor to ensure that there is no unnecessary movement of the patient. Collars, sandbags, and splints are not always radiolucent, and it may be necessary to remove them once preliminary films have been obtained. Riggins found that there was no radiological evidence of trauma in 17% of adult patients with spinal cord injury.[1] When in doubt seek a radiological opinion, especially with radiographs of children, which are difficult to assess and are often normal in spinal cord injury.

Cervical spine

In a patient with multiple trauma radiographs of the cervical spine, chest, and pelvis are mandatory. If there is depression of consciousness skull radiographs or a computed tomographic scan of the head (if available) are required.

Most radiologically detectable abnormalities of the neck are shown in a standard lateral radiograph, which must display all seven cervical vertebrae and the C7-T1 junction if injuries are not to be missed. This can usually be achieved by applying traction to both arms, but pain in the neck or exacerbation of neurological symptoms must be avoided. If the lower cervical vertebrae are still not adequately shown a "swimmer's view" and, if necessary, conventional or computed tomograms can be requested. These are helpful in excluding important lesions at the cervicothoracic junction.

Assessing spinal radiographs

Check
- Anterior vertebral border
- Posterior vertebral border
- Posterior facet margins
- Anterior border of spinous processes
- Posterior border of spinous processes
- Integrity of vertebral bodies, laminae, pedicles, and arches
- Prevertebral space
- Interspinous gaps
- For rotational deformity
- All three basic views of cervical spine and two of thoracolumbar spine
- Lateral view of sternum (for unstable thoracic injury)

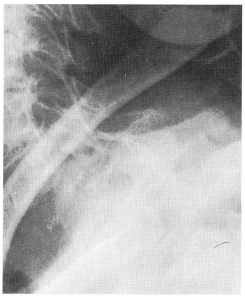

Swimmer's view showing dislocation of C6 on C7.

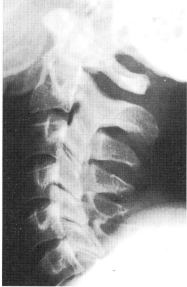
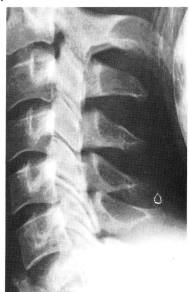

Compression fracture of C7, missed initially because of failure to show the entire cervical spine.

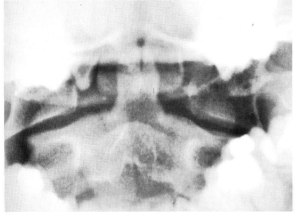

Open mouth odontoid view showing a Jefferson fracture of the atlas with outward displacement of the right lateral mass.

The lateral radiograph will normally show fractures, subluxations, and dislocations. Unilateral facet dislocation is associated with forward vertebral displacement of less than half the diameter of the vertebral body. This produces a change in the rotational orientation of the spine at the level of injury. Displacement of more than half the vertebral width normally indicates bilateral facet dislocation.

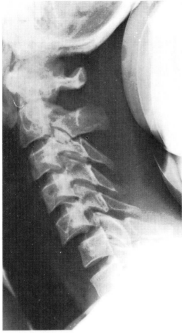

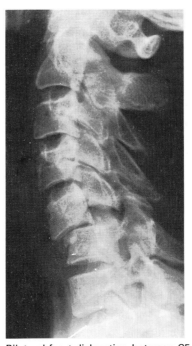

Unilateral facet dislocation between C5 and C6.

Bilateral facet dislocation between C5 and C6.

Many patients present with more subtle signs of an unstable injury. A chip fracture of the lower and anterior margin of the vertebra ("tear drop" fracture) is commonly associated with an unstable flexion injury. This may produce widening of the interspinous gap, loss of normal cervical lordosis, and minor subluxation. Always look for a prevertebral haematoma, which is indicated by an increased gap between the nasopharynx or trachea and cervical spine. The retropharyngeal space (C2) should not exceed 7 mm in adults or children, whereas the retrotracheal space (C6) should not exceed 22 mm in adults or 14 mm in children. (The retropharyngeal space widens in a crying child.)

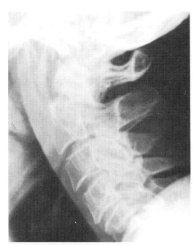

Odontoid fracture with posterior displacement of the anterior arch of the atlas.

The other standard radiographs of the cervical spine are the open mouth odontoid view and the anteroposterior projection. Abnormalities are more likely to be seen in the odontoid radiograph (for example, Jefferson fractures of the atlas as well as odontoid fractures), but the odontoid and atlantoaxial joints must not be obscured by overlying teeth. In the anteroposterior radiograph look closely at the upper thoracic vertebrae and the first two ribs. Also take care to examine the alignment of spinous processes, which may be displaced laterally at sites of unilateral facet dislocation.

When standard radiographs are normal but cervical injury is suspected flexion and extension radiographs may be obtained later as long as neurological symptoms and signs are absent. Even these radiographs, however, may show no evidence of instability in children with cord injury or adults with cord compression resulting from spondylosis or acute disc prolapse. Rupture of the transverse ligament of the atlas is associated with an increased atlanto-odontoid gap, which should not normally exceed 3 mm in adults and 5 mm in children.

Supine oblique radiographs of the cervical spine help to confirm the presence of facet dislocation if standard radiographs are difficult to interpret, particularly those of the cervicothoracic junction.

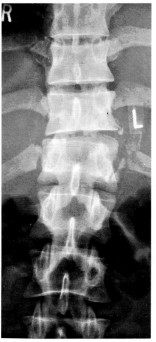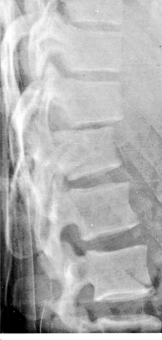

Fracture dislocation of T11 on T12.

Thoracolumbar spine

Anteroposterior and lateral radiographs are the standard radiographs of the thoracolumbar spine. Unlike a cervical haematoma a paravertebral haematoma in the thoracolumbar region is best seen on an anteroposterior radiograph, in which it may be responsible for mediastinal widening that resembles aortic dissection. In the lateral radiograph particular importance should be attached to subluxation, burst fractures, or potentially unstable injury affecting the posterior vertebral ligaments or bone (laminae and pedicles). Instability requires at least two of the three columns of the spine to be disrupted.[2] The upper thoracic spine is usually difficult to assess in the lateral radiograph, and if symptoms or signs indicate, tomograms or computed tomograms should be considered.

Injuries of the thoracic spine can be rendered unstable by fractures of the ribs and sternum, which must be examined by radiography. An appreciable force is required to produce an unstable thoracic injury, which is usually evident in the standard radiographs.

Treatment

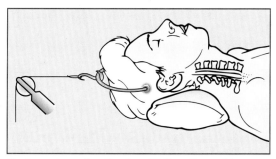

Skull traction using Gardner-Wells caliper with neck roll in position to maintain postural reduction.

Cervical injuries

At the district hospital orthopaedic surgeons should participate in the patient's management at an early stage. Unstable cervical injuries may be immobilised by a firm collar or skeletal traction. No technique is foolproof, and treatment should be supervised by a senior member of the medical staff. Skull traction helps to correct the alignment of the injured spine, reduce fractures and dislocations, decompress the cord and nerve roots, and provide stability.

Various skull calipers are available, but spring loaded types such as the Gardner-Wells calipers are easily applied and carry a low risk of complications. In recent years halo traction has become more popular as it may be converted to a halo brace to allow the patient to mobilise. Care must be taken not to overdistract injuries of the upper cervical spine, and for some of these traction is contraindicated. For interhospital transfer, immobilisation of the head with a semirigid collar, sandbags and tape provides effective spinal protection.

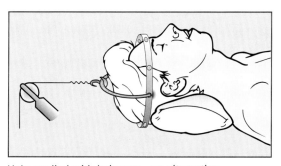

Halo applied with bale arm—an alternative approach to skull traction if early mobilisation into a halo brace is being considered.

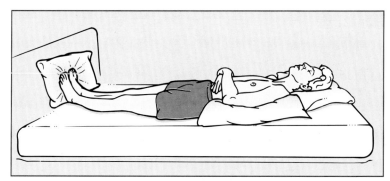

Conservative treatment for thoracolumbar injuries (postural reduction).

Thoracolumbar injuries

Thoracolumbar injuries may be treated by "postural reduction", which entails bed rest on a lumbar support to maintain the normal lordosis and help reduce the fracture or dislocation. Doctors commonly operate on patients with unstable injuries to enable them to be mobilised without much delay and to facilitate nursing care, though this approach is controversial.

Spine and spinal cord

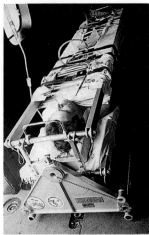

Patient immobilised in a Royal Air Force pattern turning frame for transfer to a spinal injury unit. Skull traction is maintained by means of the constant tension device.

Spinal injury associated with paraplegia or tetraplegia

Because of the medical complications associated with paraplegia or tetraplegia early referral and transfer to a spinal centre allows the patient to receive better overall care. Many spinal centres have intensive care units, and staff are experienced in dealing with complicated cases. Referral should be the responsibility of the orthopaedic or neurosurgical team. Routine administration of mannitol and antibiotics in these patients is of no proved benefit. However, the second national acute spinal cord injury study in the United States has shown that the degree of neurological injury may be reduced if very high doses of steroids are given during the first 24 hours after injury.[3] A policy should be agreed with the local spinal injury centre. There is no conclusive evidence that surgery improves neurological outcome, but it is undertaken when there are signs of deteriorating neurological function and also to prevent deformity. The prognosis is always uncertain, and patients should therefore be treated actively. Magnetic resonance imaging is now the investigation of choice for visualising the spinal cord, assessing the extent of injury, and guiding the prognosis.

Drug treatment in spinal cord injury

Consult your spinal unit for advice. Aim to give methylprednisolone at the earliest opportunity: 30 mg/kg intravenously over 15 minutes and then 5.4 mg/kg/h for 23 hours

1 Riggins R. The risk of neurologic damage with fractures of the vertebrae. *J Trauma* 1977;**17**:126–33.
2 Denis F. Thoracolumbar spinal injuries: classification. *Current Orthopaedics* 1988; **2**: 214–17.
3 Bracken MB, Shepard MJ, Collins WF, *et al*. A randomized, controlled trial of methylprednisolone or naloxone in the treatment of acute spinal cord injury: results of the second national acute spinal cord injury study. *N Engl J Med* 1990;**322**:1405–11.

9 ABDOMEN

Andrew Cope, William Stebbings

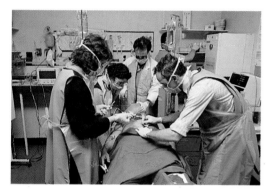

The aim of this chapter is to enable all those concerned with the management of patients with abdominal trauma to perform a thorough examination and assessment with the help of diagnostic tests and to institute safe and correct treatment.

Intra-abdominal injuries carry a high morbidity and mortality because they are often not detected or their severity is underestimated. This is particularly common in cases of blunt trauma, in which there may be few or no external signs. Always have a high index of suspicion of abdominal injury when the history suggests severe trauma. Traditionally, abdominal trauma is classified as either blunt or penetrating, but the initial assessment and, if required, resuscitation are essentially the same.

Blunt trauma

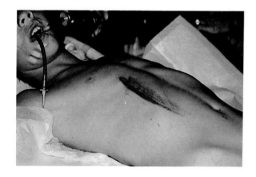

Road traffic accidents are one of the commonest causes of blunt injuries. Since wearing seat belts was made compulsory the number of fatal head injuries has declined, but a pattern of blunt abdominal trauma that is specific to seat belts has emerged. This often includes avulsion injuries of the mesentery of the small bowel. The symptoms and signs of blunt abdominal trauma can be subtle, and consequently diagnosis is difficult. A high degree of suspicion of underlying intra-abdominal injury must be adopted when dealing with blunt trauma. Blunt abdominal trauma is usually associated with trauma to other areas, especially the head, chest, and pelvis.

Penetrating trauma

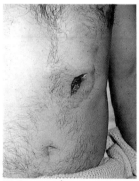
Stab wound.

Penetrating wounds are either due to low velocity projectiles such as knives or hand gun bullets or high velocity projectiles such as rifle bullets and shrapnel from bombs or blasts. With the increasing prevalence of civilian violence penetrating injuries, especially those due to stabbing, are encountered increasingly in accident and emergency departments. Visceral injury occurs in 80%–90% of bullet wounds but only 30% of stab wounds. Penetrating wounds may seem easy to diagnose, but it is difficult to assess whether peritoneal penetration has occurred. About a third of abdominal stab wounds with serious visceral injury at operation have minimal physical signs.

Assessment

> **Remember the A, B, C of the primary survey**

> **To evaluate the abdomen Look, Feel, and Listen**

Doctors must perform the primary survey—namely, airway management with protection of the cervical spine, breathing, circulatory and initial neurological evaluation. The circulation may be compromised if there is concealed intra-abdominal bleeding. The usual diagnostic pathway of taking the history, physical examination, and special investigations cannot always be followed as resuscitation is the highest priority. The sequence of look, feel, and listen will help in the rapid initial evaluation of the abdomen.

Procedure

Information required in patients with abdominal trauma

From the patient or relatives and friends:
- History of allergies
- History of alcohol or drug misuse
- Medical history
- Current medication

From the police and ambulance crew:
- Speed of the vehicle
- Nature and direction of impact
- Evidence of deformation of the vehicle
- Evidence of steering wheel injury
- Whether a seat belt was worn
- Injuries to other victims

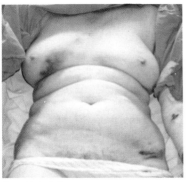

Seat belt injury.

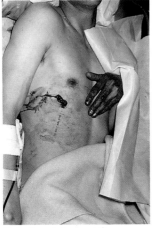

Anterior stab wound.

Signs of urethral injury

Blood at external meatus

High riding prostate

Bruised scrotum

Bruised perineum

Take a careful history

The patient may have limited recall of the injury owing to loss of consciousness, alcohol intoxication, or hysteria. Relatives and friends can provide information regarding medical conditions, current drugs, allergies, and alcohol or drug misuse.

In victims of road traffic accidents further information on the type of injury with regard to the speed of the vehicle, the nature of the impact, evidence of a steering wheel injury, whether seat belts were worn, and the condition of the other victims should be sought from the police and ambulance crews.

Useful information in patients with penetrating injuries includes their position when shot or stabbed and the length of the blade or the type of gun and the number and range of shots fired.

Perform a thorough examination

Look—You cannot perform an adequate assessment without exposing the patient fully; therefore you must remove all of the patient's clothes. Look systematically at the anterior structures, including the urethral meatus in men, the flanks, and the posterior structures—the back, buttocks, and perineum—for bruises, lacerations, entry and exit wounds, and impressions of seat belts or tyres. Any abnormality should be recorded.

Feel—Palpation, both superficial and deep, should include all abdominal structures. The abdomen starts at the level of the fifth rib, and therefore penetrating wounds of the lower chest can enter the abdominal cavity. The assessment of blunt trauma is difficult. Muscle guarding resulting from intraperitoneal injury but can also be due to injury to the abdominal wall. Signs of peritoneal irritation after rupture of a hollow viscus can be slow to develop, and consequently the physical signs must be re-evaluated repeatedly. Abdominal rigidity usually indicates visceral injury; percussion and tenderness on coughing are also useful indicators of intraperitoneal injury. Instability of the pelvic ring can be confirmed by applying direct pressure in two planes to both anterior superior iliac spines. The superior pubic rami should be palpated in addition to the symphysis. Retroperitoneal injuries are difficult to diagnose but should be considered if there is a spinal deformity or paravertebral haematoma or if the mechanism of the injury suggests possible damage to retroperitoneal structures.

Listen—The presence or absence of bowel sounds and their quality if present should be recorded. The presence of bowel sounds does not exclude major peritoneal injury.

Rectal examination—Rectal examination is essential. Loss of integrity of the rectal wall and the presence of blood indicate trauma of the large bowel; a high lying prostate indicates urethral damage.

Vaginal examination—Disruption of the pubic rami or symphysis may cause vaginal injury, therefore, vaginal examination is mandatory, not only to confirm the integrity of the vaginal wall but also to detect obvious pelvic fractures, particularly of the inferior rami.

Examination of urethral meatus—In men the meatus should be examined for evidence of urethral injury. If there is blood at the meatus a urethral catheter should not be passed, and a urologist's opinion should be requested.

The doctor must ensure that airway management with protection of the cervical spine, breathing, and circulation are adequate before proceeding to the special investigations.

Special investigations

Baseline blood tests

- Send a blood sample for cross matching, specifying the number of units required
- Measure haemoglobin concentration, white cell count, and packed cell volume
- Measure serum urea and electrolyte concentrations, serum amylase activity, and arterial blood gas tensions

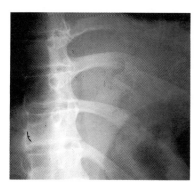

Fractures of the 10th and 11th ribs.

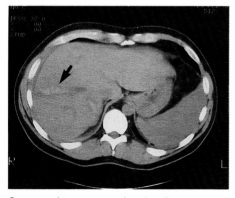

Computed tomogram showing liver laceration.

Perform baseline tests

Determination of baseline haemoglobin concentration, white cell count, packed cell volume, and cross matching is essential in all victims of trauma. Blood for these tests may be obtained while an intravenous cannula of gauge 14 is being inserted. As a general rule it is safer to overestimate the amount of cross matched blood required. Biochemical measurements that should be made include urea and electrolyte concentrations, serum amylase activity, and blood gas tensions.

Pass a nasogastric tube

A nasogastric tube will not only empty the stomach contents but may also suggest upper gastrointestinal injury if blood is aspirated. The tube should be passed orally if there is a suggestion of a fracture of the cribriform plate.

Insert a urethral catheter

A urethral catheter is mandatory in all patients with severe trauma except those in whom urethral injury is suspected, when the suprapubic route should be used.

Perform radiography of the chest and abdomen

An erect chest radiograph is preferable to a supine abdominal film for excluding the possibility of free intraperitoneal air. Abdominal radiographs may show fractures of lower ribs, which may be the only sign of intra-abdominal damage, or fractures of the transverse processes, which may suggest ureteric injury. They can also confirm the presence of opaque foreign bodies (for example, bullets), confirm the position of the nasogastric tube, and show acute gastric dilatation.

In multisystem trauma radiography of the lateral cervical spine and pelvis is also performed.

Additional imaging

Imaging techniques such as ultrasonography and computed tomography are not usually available for routine diagnosis in an accident and emergency department. Centres that have portable ultrasonic facilities should consider using them to assess possible subcapsular splenic haematomas or renal injuries. They should be used only after initial stabilisation and when there is no indication for immediate laparotomy. Computed tomography is valuable in diagnosing pancreatic and other retroperitoneal injuries.

Indications for laparotomy

Indications for laparotomy

- Unexplained shock
- Rigid silent abdomen
- Evisceration
- Radiological evidence of free intraperitoneal gas
- Radiological evidence of ruptured diaphragm
- All gunshot wounds
- Positive result of peritoneal lavage

If laparotomy is to be performed notify the most senior surgeon present and the anaesthetist immediately and alert the staff of the operating theatre.

Urgent laparotomy is required for profound hypovolaemia due to haemorrhage that persists despite adequate replacement of fluid volume when there is no overt cause (for example, haemothorax or a pelvic fracture).

Peritoneal lavage

If there is no indication for an urgent laparotomy peritoneal lavage may help decide which patients subsequently require surgical assessment by laparotomy.

Contraindications

The only absolute contraindication for lavage is if there is already an indication for urgent laparotomy. Relative contraindications are pregnancy, gross obesity, coagulopathy, and previous lower abdominal surgery.

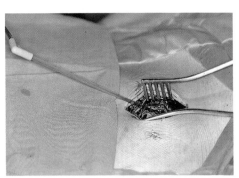

Peritoneal lavage.

Procedure

(1) Explain the procedure to the patient if he or she is conscious

(2) Ensure that a urethral or suprapubic catheter and a nasogastric tube are in place

(3) Prepare the patient's abdominal skin with antiseptic, and drape sterile towels over the abdomen

(4) Infiltrate the skin with a solution of 1% lignocaine and 1 in 200 000 adrenaline

(5) Make a vertical subumbilical incision in the midline 5 cm in length centred at one third of the distance between the umbilicus and the symphysis pubis

(6) Under direct vision divide the linea alba and identify the peritoneum

(7) Make an incision into the peritoneum and insert a peritoneal dialysis catheter (without an introducer) towards the pelvis

(8) Aspirate any free blood or enteric contents. If more than 5 ml of blood is aspirated an urgent laparotomy is indicated

(9) If no blood is aspirated infuse 1 litre of warm (37 °C) physiological saline

(10) Allow the saline to equilibrate for three minutes and then place the bag and giving set on the floor with the tap open and drain as much of the original 1 litre as possible

(11) Send a 20 ml sample to the laboratory for measurement of white and red blood cell counts and for microscopic examination.

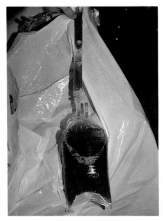

Bag and giving set after drainage of saline. The result was positive.

Interpretation of results

If >5 ml of blood or enteric contents is aspirated laparotomy is mandatory. If fluid from peritoneal lavage is obtained from either the urinary catheter or a chest drain an urgent laparotomy is essential.

Patients with a positive result must have a laparotomy. Patients with a negative result may be managed conservatively and should be frequently re-examined by the surgeon responsible for the patient.

False positive results occur in about 2% of cases, particularly when the lavage is performed blind, and are caused either by trauma to vessels in the abdominal wall or by perforating a viscus with the trochar.

False negative results also occur in about 2% of cases. Most of these are thought to be attributable to injury to retroperitoneal structures and, occasionally, to diaphragmatic injuries.

Considerations for management

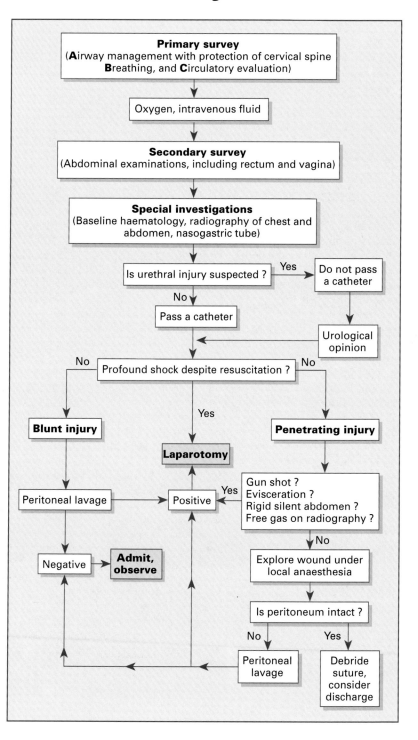

Penetrating trauma

All patients with gunshot wounds, regardless of the muzzle velocity of the gun, must have a laparotomy.

The tracks of stab wounds should be explored (not probed) to show the integrity of the peritoneum. If the peritoneum is not intact a laparotomy should be considered.

Lower chest wounds can be managed conservatively with careful monitoring, assuming that the results of lavage are negative.

Flank and back wounds are difficult to assess even with the aid of peritoneal lavage, ultrasonography, or computed tomography, and therefore laparotomy should be considered.

Evisceration of bowel necessitates laparotomy.

Blunt trauma

In all cases of blunt trauma a high index of suspicion of intra-abdominal injury is essential. Blunt trauma is more difficult to assess clinically than penetrating trauma, and therefore diagnostic peritoneal lavage is helpful in evaluating the need for laparotomy.

If laparotomy is not indicated initially

Consider admission for all patients with suspected intra-abdominal injuries so that re-evaluation and observation including of vital signs can continue. Such admissions will normally be to the general surgical ward, unless the patient's other injuries require intensive care.

Conclusion

Abdominal injuries should never be underestimated. In a recent retrospective study of 1000 deaths due to injury 43% of the deaths not related to the central nervous system were judged to have been potentially preventable. Among the commonest missed diagnoses were those of ruptured liver and ruptured spleen.[1] Thorough initial assessment and repeated re-evaluation with appropriate investigations are of prime importance for detecting these injuries.

1 Anderson ID, Woodford M, de Dombal T, Irving M. Retrospective study of 1000 deaths from injury in England and Wales. *BMJ* 1988;**296**:1305–8.

10 THE URINARY TRACT

Timothy Terry, Anthony Deane

UPPER URINARY TRACT

Typical victims of urinary tract trauma

Young men while performing a sporting activity (55% of cases)

People in road traffic accidents (25% of cases)

Victims of domestic or industrial accidents (15% of cases)

Victims of assault (5% of cases)

In the United Kingdom over 90% of renal injuries are a result of blunt abdominal trauma. Important associated injuries occur in about 40% of patients with blunt renal trauma. A high index of suspicion of a renal lesion is required in the patient with multiple injuries as the signs and symptoms of the renal trauma may be obscured by those of the concomitant injuries.

In children the kidney is the organ most commonly injured by blunt abdominal trauma. This may be explained by the relative lack of perinephric fat in children and the incidence (of up to 20%) of pre-existing renal abnormalities (primary pelviureteric junction obstruction is the commonest).

The mechanism of renal injury due to blunt abdominal trauma may be direct or indirect. With a direct injury the kidney is either crushed between the anterior end of the 12th rib and the lumbar spine—such as in sporting injuries—or between an external force applied to the abdomen anteriorly just below the rib cage and the paravertebral muscles—such as in run over accidents and injuries caused by seat belts and steering columns. Indirect injury occurs when a deceleration force is applied to the renal pedicle (as a result of falling from a height and landing on the buttocks). Such injuries can tear the major renal vessels or rupture the ureter at the pelviureteric junction.

Penetrating renal trauma occurs in about 7% of patients with abdominal stab wounds. As with blunt renal trauma associated injuries are often present (in up to 80% of cases); these affect the liver, lungs, spleen, small bowel, stomach, pancreas, duodenum, and diaphragm in descending order of frequency. Renal stab wounds are potentially serious, with the possibilities of severed major renal vessels and lacerations to the collecting system or upper ureter. Gunshot wounds that involve the kidney may be caused by a low or high velocity missile. Low velocity missiles cause injury by directly penetrating the tissue whereas high velocity missiles produce direct tissue injury plus damage to adjacent tissue because of the shock wave effect (see chapter 24).

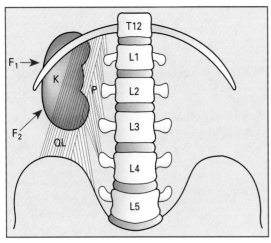

Mechanism of direct blunt renal trauma. An external force (F₁) may crush the kidney (K) between the 12th rib and the vertebral column, or a force (F₂) may crush the kidney against the paravertebral muscles (quadratus lumborum (QL) or psoas major in position P but deleted from diagram).

Classification of renal trauma

Classification of renal injuries

Minor (85%)
- Contusions
- Superficial lacerations (capsule and pelvicaliceal system intact)

Major (10%)
- Deep lacerations (capsular tears or pelvicaliceal involvement, or both)

Critical (5%)
- Renal fragmentation
- Pedicle injuries (renal artery thrombosis, vessel avulsion, and pelviureteric rupture)

Renal injuries can be classified as minor, major, or critical, based on the clinical and radiological assessments of the patient. Minor injuries (contusions and superficial lacerations) consist of parenchymal damage without capsular tears or involvement of the pelvicaliceal system. Major injuries (deep lacerations) consist of parenchymal damage with capsular tears or extension into the collecting system, or both. Critical injuries include kidney fragmentation and injuries to the pedicle (such as renal artery thrombosis, avulsion of renal vessels, and rupture of the pelviureteric junction).

Clinical presentation

Clinical signs of renal trauma

- Regional skin lesions (abrasions, bruising, and entry and exit wounds)
- Loin tenderness
- Loss of loin contour
- Loin mass
- Gross haematuria (up to 90% of cases)

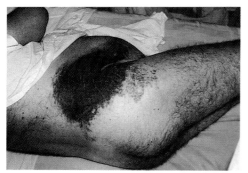

Severe abdominal and flank ecchymosis with potential urological injury (caused by a seat belt).

Most patients (80%–90%) with direct renal trauma give a history of a blow to the flank and complain of loin pain, which is followed after a variable period by gross haematuria. The haematuria may be subsequently accompanied by ureteric colic caused by the passage of blood clots. Clinical examination may show skin abrasions or bruising overlying the upper abdomen, loin, or lower thoracic area. Rigidity of the anterior abdominal wall and local loin tenderness over the affected kidney are invariably elicited. A flattening of loin contour together with a palpable loin mass indicate the presence of a perinephric haematoma with or without urinary extravasation of contrast dye. In such cases a paralytic ileus may be present. Varying degrees of hypovolaemic shock may be present, but this is usually secondary to associated injuries.

About 70% of potentially lethal injuries to the renal pedicle (indirect trauma) do not cause gross haematuria. Patients with such injuries are usually in severe shock, having been brought to hospital after a fall from a height. The same mechanism, in a milder form, usually produces intimal tearings of the renal vessels, which can lead to thrombosis.

The victim of a penetrating renal injury caused by a low velocity missile or stab wound will have an obvious entrance wound. The depth and direction of the wound track and the site of the exit wound, when present, suggest the likelihood of renal involvement.

Radiological investigations

Findings on intravenous urography

Control film
- Fractures (of lower ribs and transverse processes of lumbar vertebrae)
- Loss of psoas shadow
- Loss of renal outline
- Loin mass (displacement of bowel or diaphragm

Postcontrast film series
- Distortion of caliceal pattern
- Contrast extravasation
- Non-visualisation of part or whole of caliceal system

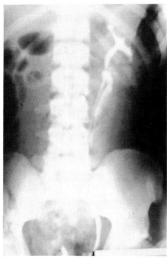

Excretory urogram with extravasation of dye.

The standard investigation in patients suspected of having a serious renal injury is intravenous urography. This includes all patients with gross haematuria and those with microscopic haematuria and a systolic blood pressure <90 mm Hg. Haemodynamically stable patients with microscopic haematuria have minor renal injuries and do not require urography.

The preliminary control film shows abnormalities in about 15% of patients with blunt renal trauma. These abnormalities include pneumothorax or haemothorax; concomitant fractures of ribs and the transverse processes of lumbar vertebrae; scoliosis with concavity towards the side of injury; loss of psoas shadow or renal outline due to perirenal haematoma; a soft tissue loin mass displacing bowel shadows or raising the ipsilateral hemidiaphragm; and free intraperitoneal gas. In 85% of patients with blunt renal trauma the postcontrast series of radiographs shows no abnormalities. The appearances in the remainder are those of distortion of caliceal pattern, extravasation of contrast dye into the perinephric tissues, or failure to visualise any part or the whole of the caliceal system. These findings suggest the presence of a major or critical renal injury, and the appearance in the intravenous urogram of a normal contralateral kidney is reassuring.

If patients with blunt trauma are clinically stable further information on the precise state of the damaged kidney (the presence of parenchymal disruption, intrarenal or subcapsular haematomas, and perirenal collections) may be gained by renal ultrasonography. This technique is particularly valuable for imaging injuries to the kidneys that are not visualised in the urogram and for following the natural course of perirenal collections. Computed tomography with enhancement with an intravenous radiocontrast agent, although a popular technique for investigating blunt abdominal trauma, is unlikely to give any additional information in patients with renal trauma over that provided by intravenous urography with nephrotomography and complemented with ultrasonography. Selective renal arteriography is indicated in patients with vascular pedicle injuries whose condition is stable and in patients with macroscopic haematuria persisting longer than one week. In the rare cases in which the mode of the accident and the findings on urography suggest the possibility of disruption of the pelviureteric junction a retrograde ureterogram is necessary.

Management

The principle underlying the management of patients with renal trauma is conservation of the maximum number of functioning nephrons with minimal morbidity and mortality. The immediate management of any individual patient is determined, however, more by the patient's general clinical state and the presence of important associated injuries than by the mode and type of renal injury. Less than 5% of all renal injuries are by themselves life threatening, and hypovolaemic shock in a patient with renal trauma is nearly always secondary to the presence of concomitant injuries. The initial general clinical assessment of the patient is thus all important in deciding a plan of supportive and definitive treatment.

In patients with blunt renal trauma urgent surgical exploration for critical injuries (renal fragmentation and pedicle injuries) is mandatory. A generous midline abdominal incision allows complete assessment of the abdomen for concomitant injuries while providing access to the entire length of both ureters, the kidneys, and the vascular pedicles. If conservative renal surgery is being contemplated the ipsilateral renal vessels must be isolated and controlled before Gerota's fascia is incised. Partial nephrectomy may be possible in some patients with fragmented kidneys, but usually total nephrectomy is necessary. Lacerations to the major renal vein may be debrided and sutured. If renal artery thrombosis has been diagnosed within 6 hours of injury, thrombectomy, excision of the damaged arterial segment, and direct end to end reanastomosis may be considered.

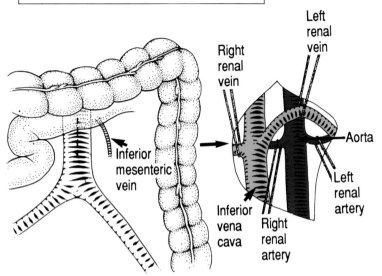

(Left) Retroperitoneal incision sited over the aorta medial to the inferior mesenteric vein to isolate the renal vessels before opening Gerota's fascia. (Right) The left renal vein crosses anterior to the aorta. With this vein retracted superiorly the left and right renal arteries may be located arising from the aorta.

Disruption of the pelviureteric junction is treated by spatulation of the ends and reanastomosis over a ureteric stent.

Minor renal injuries (contusions and superficial lacerations) and major injuries (deep lacerations), which together comprise about 95% of cases of closed renal trauma, are initially managed expectantly. Strict bed rest, appropriate analgesia, and prophylactic antibiotics (cephradine or trimethoprim) are instituted together with frequent serial clinical observations of vital signs and assessment of any loin swelling. Once the vital signs are stable ambulation is allowed only after gross haematuria has cleared (serial aliquots of urine are kept for comparison) and the perirenal swelling, if present, has clinically resolved.

Whether to perform early surgery in patients with major renal injuries is a controversial issue, but it is clearly indicated in those rare cases in which primary haemorrhage or secondary haemorrhage at 10–14 days, usually due to infection, endangers life. The late complications (after six weeks) of major renal injuries that may require surgery include hypertension, arteriovenous fistula, hydronephrosis, formation of pseudocysts or calculi, chronic pyelonephritis, and loss of renal function. Regular follow up is necessary in patients with major renal trauma during the first year after injury if these late complications, of which hypertension is the most common, are not to be missed.

Most penetrating renal stab wounds and all gunshot wounds involving the upper urinary tract require immediate surgical exploration to exclude or treat associated injuries, to assess and repair renal or ureteric damage, and to allow wound debridement.

Finally, an unsuspected penetrating or blunt renal injury may manifest itself at emergency laparotomy performed to control massive intra-abdominal bleeding in a patient with trauma. The clinically silent renal injury manifests itself as a retroperitoneal haematoma. In such cases on table intravenous urography is essential to establish the presence of a normal functioning contralateral kidney and to determine the type of injury to the damaged kidney. The retroperitoneal haematoma should be explored only if a critical injury is identified in the urogram or if the haematoma is large and is seen to expand during laparotomy. In either case the renal vessels must be controlled before opening Gerota's fascia, otherwise the possible use of conservative renal surgery may be jeopardised.

LOWER URINARY TRACT

Investigations in patients with lower urinary tract injuries

- Inspect the urinary meatus for blood
- Examine the abdomen for peritonism, perineal bruising, and a high riding prostate
- Perform intravenous urography to detect bladder perforation, displaced bladder, upper urinary tract injury

Perform cystography to exclude bladder perforation if patient has a catheter in place

Perform ascending urethrography (aqueous contrast) to exclude urethral injury (controversial)

Injuries of the lower urinary tract cause more confusion than those of the upper urinary tract as their management is controversial. The rule in patients with suspected urethral injuries and major pelvic fractures is not to pass a urethral catheter without first seeking advice from a urologist. Even though monitoring urinary output is very important in patients with major injuries, a catheter should not be passed without careful thought. Urinary extravasation is not dangerous in the short term.

Bladder injuries

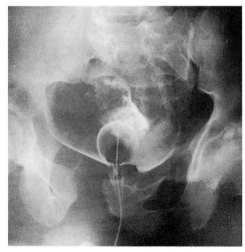

Cystogram of a bladder full of haematoma with extravasation of contrast due to a torn anterior bladder wall. The patient required 30 units of blood before bleeding was controlled by selective internal iliac embolisation.

Bladder injuries may be associated with a pelvic fracture—that is, they may be caused by penetration by a bony fragment or by a direct blow to the lower abdomen, especially when the bladder is full. The condition may be missed in patients intoxicated with alcohol or those with a head injury. Patients with a bladder injury may have lower abdominal peritonism and not be able to pass urine. A catheter may have been passed by the receiving clinicians and the urine may contain blood.

Investigation begins by inspecting the plain radiograph to exclude pelvic fractures. Disruption of the pelvic symphysis alerts the clinician to the possibility of urethral injury and delayed rupture of the bladder due to stretching of the anterior bladder wall. An intravenous urogram may show an extravasation from a bladder injury. If there is no pelvic fracture and no urethral haemorrhage a urethral catheter may be passed, and cystography with 10% dilute contrast agent will show any important bladder injury. If an intraperitoneal bladder rupture is suspected then cystography should be done before diagnostic peritoneal lavage because a laparotomy will be required to repair such a lesion, if it is present, making lavage unnecessary. In patients with serious pelvic fracture, especially if it affects the pubic symphysis, upward dislocation of the bladder on urography should be excluded first, although this would usually be accompanied by urethral haemorrhage.

Treatment—Patients with important intraperitoneal ruptures with peritonism are best treated by laparotomy and drainage by suprapubic catheter as well as by urethral catheter for about seven days. Broad range antibiotics should be given. Extraperitoneal injuries are managed by drainage by catheter without irrigation for about 10 days. A catheter of at least 20 FG is necessary, and cystography to confirm healing is advisable before withdrawal of the catheter.

Bulbar injuries

Management of patients with bulbar injuries

- Do not pass a urethral catheter
- If the patient passes urine give antibiotics and follow up
- If the patient has urinary retention insert a suprapubic catheter with a small calibre and give antibiotics. Perform urethrography after about five days and follow up

Bulbar injuries occur by direct trauma—for example, by falling on to a bicycle crossbar. Occasionally they can be caused by penetrating trauma. Patients with bulbar injuries have perineal bruising and blood at the urinary meatus. A urethral catheter must not be passed as it may aggravate the injury and introduce infection. The patient should be treated expectantly, and, if he or she passes urine, should be given antibiotics and followed up. Patients with urinary retention should be treated by inserting a suprapubic catheter with a small calibre percutaneously as heavy haematuria is not usually a problem. Antibiotics are given, and urethrography can be performed after about five days. The patient will need urological follow up to exclude the formation of a stricture.

Urethral injuries caused by pelvic fracture

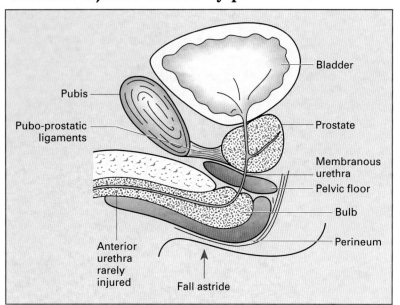

The puboprostatic ligaments carry the prostate with them in patients with pelvic fracture, tearing the urethra off the pelvic floor.

The membranous urethra below the prostate is damaged in about 10% of men with pelvic fractures. Serious injuries, though rare, are devastating as impotence and stricture are common sequels. Damage usually comprises a partial tear, but, occasionally, complete disruption and upward dislocation of the bladder and prostate occurs. The prostate is fixed to the pubic symphysis by the puboprostatic ligaments, and any severe disruption of the pubic symphysis is liable to tear the prostate off the membranous urethra, which is attached to the pelvic floor.

Signs of membranous urethral injury

- Pelvic fracture
- Perineal bruising
- Blood at the meatus
- Inability to pass urine
- High riding prostate

The signs of urethral injury caused by pelvic fracture are blood at the meatus, perineal bruising, and inability to pass urine. A urethral catheter must not be passed as it may aggravate the injury, even if it passes the tear: the urethra is often traumatised and devascularised and may be eroded by the catheter or disintegrate around it; the catheter will prevent the haematoma from draining and introduce infection with possible fistulation on its withdrawal; and worst of all, the catheter may pass out of the tear and drain blood and urine below the prostate. Balloon inflation may convert a partial disruption into a complete one.

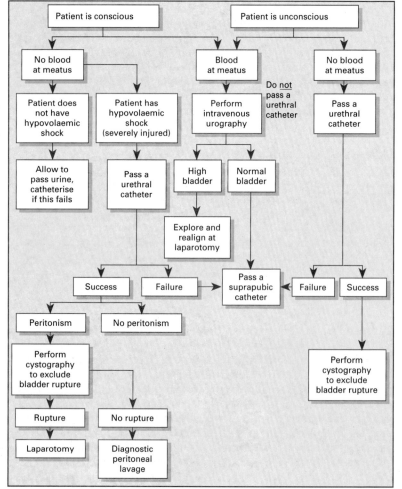

Urological management of men with serious pelvic fractures.

The safest way to treat urethral injuries caused by pelvic fracture is to pass a suprapubic catheter of adequate calibre either percutaneously or by cystotomy if the patient requires a laparotomy for other reasons or if the bladder is impalpable. Intravenous urography should be performed to exclude total disruption with a high riding bladder above the pubic symphysis—an indication for exploration and repositioning. Some authorities advise performing ascending urethrography to delineate the extent of the injury and plan its management, but this can be difficult in the emergency room. In general a urethral catheter can be passed in a patient with a pelvic fracture if there is no blood at the meatus or if the pubic symphysis is not severely disrupted on radiography. If any difficulties are encountered urological help should be summoned and an ascending urethrogram considered or suprapubic catheterisation performed. If there is severe disruption of the pubic symphysis orthopaedic help should be requested as early fixation may assist in management and reduce morbidity. Later treatment of these injuries entails urethroscopy, but late strictures are very common.

In women the urethra is injured only rarely, and usually a catheter can easily be passed in those with pelvic fractures and, if necessary, cystography performed to exclude the possibility of bladder injuries.

External genitalia

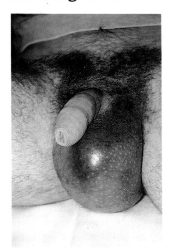

Scrotal haematoma.

Serious injuries to the penis and scrotum are unusual. The mobile scrotal skin can be used to cover penile defects and has good powers of recovery. Scrotal tears heal well without suturing. The erectile mechanism should always be repaired if torn with monofilament non-absorbable sutures.

The testicles can be damaged by direct trauma—usually a blow or a kick. If bleeding is confined to the scrotal skin no active treatment is required. Tense haematoceles should, however, always be explored as these usually indicate that the testis is torn and needs repair. Severe damage may require orchidectomy.

11   LIMB INJURIES

Keith M Willett, Raymond Ross, Hugh Dorrell, Peter Kelly

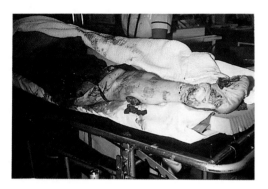

Up to 70% of multiply injured patients have injured limbs and fractures or dislocations of the appendicular skeleton. Severe limb injuries must not distract the resuscitation team from the priorities of establishing an airway, optimising ventilation, and restoring circulatory volume as limb injuries are rarely immediately life threatening, except those that cause exsanguination.

Careful thorough examination, however, is required after resuscitation to identify injuries, particularly those threatening the survival of limbs or fractures whose acute management will influence overall mortality or morbidity. Apparently minor injuries must likewise not be neglected as these may result in long term disability or disfigurement.

Prehospital care

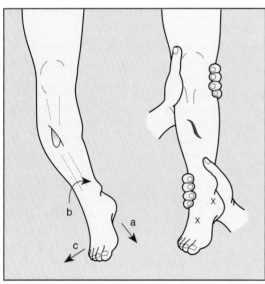

(1) Reduction of a major deformity; (a) perform gentle longitudinal traction (b) restore the correct rotation; (c) restore the alignment.
(2) Control of the fracture; check pulses (×); maintain traction; apply a splint.

Doctors attending the scene of an accident should confine themselves initially to personal safety, assessment of the scene, and management of the patient's airway, cervical spine, breathing, and circulation. Attention can then be directed towards immobilisation of the injured limbs. When moving a patient with a fractured limb the pain is reduced by supporting the limb on either side of the fracture and applying gentle traction along the axis of the limb. All unnecessary handling of the injured part without splinting should be avoided. The exceptions to this rule are when either severe deformity or ischaemia of the limb distal to the fracture threatens survival of the soft tissues; reduction is then indicated. This is achieved by gentle traction and restoration of the normal anatomical alignment. Perfusion of the distal limb must be checked after any manipulation. Prehospital care must avoid further soft tissue injury.

Splints are mandatory before the victim is evacuated, and anything rigid can be utilised—for example, pieces of wreckage, and wooden sticks. Strapping to the opposite leg is useful in solitary lower limb injuries, and "bulk" splints can be produced by bandaging blankets or pillows around the limb. Wounds should be covered with a clean dressing, preferably one that is sterile. External bleeding can be controlled by a compressive pad. Rapid transfer to hospital is then required.

Hospital care

Estimated blood loss caused by fractures

Site of fracture	Blood loss (litres)
Humerus	0·5–1·5
Tibia	0·5–1·5
Femur	1·0–2·5
Pelvis	1·0–4·0

For an open fracture the loss is two or three times greater.

Haemorrhage

Blood loss from limb wounds and occult bleeding from fractures contribute to the hypovolaemic shock in patients with multiple injuries. The accumulative haemorrhage from multiple fractures may result in exsanguination; patients with fractures of the femora and pelvis are at greatest risk. Patients with hypovolaemic shock should be resuscitated immediately with available crystalloid or colloid solutions while the dynamic response of the blood pressure and pulse is monitored. The total blood loss may be estimated (table), and blood for transfusion should be cross matched urgently. Blood loss from open fractures may be two or three times greater than that from closed fractures. Fractures, however, should not be assumed to be responsible for hypovolaemia, and occult bleeding into the visceral cavities must be excluded. Blood loss from wounds can be reduced by a compressive bandage or hand pressure over a sterile pad. A tourniquet is indicated only for unmanageable life threatening haemorrhage or after traumatic amputation.

Life threatening injuries

- Traumatic amputation
- Major vascular injury
- Pelvic fracture disruption
- Haemorrhage from open fractures
- Multiple long bone fractures
- Severe crush injury

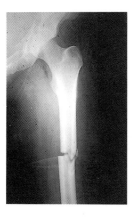

Acetabular fracture associated with a femoral shaft fracture.

Limb threatening injuries

- Vascular injury
- Major joint dislocation
- Crush injury
- Open fracture
- Compartment syndrome
- Nerve injury

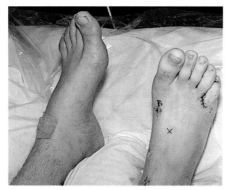

Ischaemic right foot.

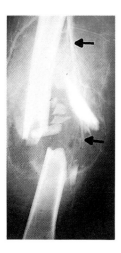

Femoral shaft fracture. Arteriogram showing occlusion of the superficial femoral artery at the level of the fracture.

Assessment

Evaluation of limb injuries is not started until the life threatening conditions have been treated. Careful examination is complemented by suspicions raised by knowledge of the mechanism of injury, information on which may be available only from attendants present at the scene of the accident. These witnesses should not be discharged until at least the mechanism, environment, time, and immediate care of the injury have been established. For victims of road traffic accidents it is important to determine whether they were a vehicle occupant, whether they were restrained by a seat belt, the direction of the impact, and the degree of damage to the vehicle. Ejection from a motor vehicle carries a high risk of serious injury.

Certain injury patterns are common. For instance, a direct blow to the knee in a seated occupant of a car may not produce only knee injury and femoral fracture but is commonly associated with hip dislocation or fractures of the acetabulum. A victim falling from a height and landing on his or her feet may sustain compression fractures of the calcaneum, ankle, tibial plateau, and one or more vertebrae at the thoracolumbar junction or in the lower cervical spine.

The patient must be completely undressed. The assessment should begin by comparing the injured limb with the uninjured limb. Observe the attitude of the limb: shortening and rotational abnormalities indicate proximal fractures or dislocations. Angular or rotational deformity may be visible or palpable. Clinical signs are often subtle, particularly in the unconscious patient, and careful inspection of the whole circumference and length of each limb for local swelling and bruising is necessary. Gently palpate along the axes of the bones and all of the surface bony prominences for tenderness, fracture crepitus (grating), and abnormal interfragmentary mobility. Carefully examine the adjacent joints so that coexisting injuries are not overlooked. A cooperative patient may indicate the active ranges of joint movement. Passive ranges of motion should be assessed cautiously in a limb that is suspected of being fractured; these should not be tested if an obvious fracture exists.

Vascular state

Of prime importance to limb survival is the competence of the vasculature distal to any injury. Local contusion, penetrating injuries, fractures, and, particularly, major joint dislocations may occlude or disrupt blood vessels. In the haemodynamically stable patient examination of the distal pulses is crucial in assessing the peripheral circulation. A diminished or absent pulse strongly suggests a vascular injury and must be explained and managed promptly. Skin colour will also indicate tissue perfusion, and pallor or a blue-grey colour should arouse suspicion. Similarly, a low skin temperature indicates inadequate perfusion. A sensitive indicator is the capillary return—the normal prompt pink flush of the nail bed seen after transient compression. This response will be slowed or blue if the circulation is inadequate.

Peripheral nerves are very sensitive to ischaemia, and sensation is lost early. Total insensibility in a hand or foot suggests ischaemia as, except in patients with injuries to the brachial plexus or spinal cord, it is unlikely that all nerve trunks will have been damaged primarily in one limb. An inadequate distal circulation is never due to spasm in a traumatised limb. If distal ischaemia is identified more proximal pulses should be checked and any major deformity at the fracture site corrected, the splint device checked for local compression, and an urgent surgical opinion sought. Dislocations of major joints require urgent reduction. Doppler ultrasonography may be useful in evaluating limb perfusion, but if a vascular injury is suspected arteriography provides the best definitive evaluation.

Limb injuries

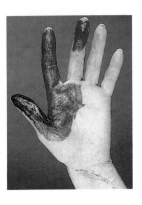

Areas of complete (black) and partial (red) sensory loss resulting from a wrist wound indicate damage to the median nerve, which was missed when the wound was sutured.

Neurological state

Evidence of nerve injury may be difficult to obtain in the unconscious or multiply injured patient. There is a higher incidence of neurological damage with dislocations than with fractures. Simple tests of sensitivity to touch, motor function, and sweating are sufficient to determine nerve integrity. When testing distal motor function the more proximal innervation of the muscle bellies must be appreciated. Division of a peripheral nerve must be assumed to have occurred if there is altered sensation in the distribution of that nerve and a wound overlying its course. Neurological function should be documented to allow later comparison.

Wound management

Management of wounds

(1) Obtain samples for culture

(2) Give preventive antibiotics intravenously

(3) Administer tetanus immunisation if necessary

(4) Remove particulate contaminants by physical wound cleaning and irrigation

(5) Excise all devitalised tissue

(6) Take a split skin graft early from skin flaps of doubtful viability

(7) Anticipate swelling, decompress compartments, and leave wounds open

(8) Obtain early fracture stabilisation

Among patients with open fractures, 50% have multiple injuries. Correct management of wounds in the first few hours is decisive. The extent of the soft tissue damage will determine the outcome. A sterile dressing applied to an open wound at the site of the accident should not be disturbed. Definitive surgical toilet is required within six hours, and repeated examinations outside the operating theatre will considerably increase the risk of infection. Instant photography of the wound has been recommended to prevent this interference. As an adjunct to surgical toilet preventive antibiotics are indicated in patients with open fractures and contaminated wounds. A cephalosporin (for example, cefuroxime 750 mg three times a day) and gentamicin (80 mg three times a day) are appropriate and should be given intravenously for at least three days. Tetanus prophylaxis must not be forgotten and depends on the patient's previous immunisation state. An immunised patient with a contaminated wound that is prone to tetanus requires a booster dose of tetanus toxoid if more than five years have elapsed since his or her last dose. In addition, tetanus immunoglobulin is required if no immunity exists or the immunisation state is unknown.

Pelvic injuries

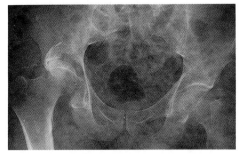

Fractured pelvis.

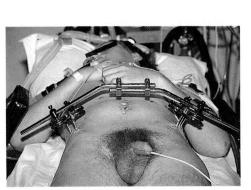

Pelvic external fixator.

Pelvic fractures must be actively sought both radiologically and clinically in all patients with multiple injuries because they are relatively common and if missed can result in catastrophic consequences. It is also important to realise that the pelvis can spring back after trauma. Consequently the displacement seen on the radiograph is usually considerably less than would have been seen at the time of impact (*see* Chapter 13). Considerable force is necessary to disrupt the pelvic ring and the associated extensive soft tissue and visceral damage may result in life-threatening haemorrhage. In these cases stabilisation of the ring with an external fixator can:

● Reduce the rate of blood loss, thereby reducing the amount of retroperitoneal haematoma, and

● Reduce the amount of soft tissue damage that would be caused by moving the patient.

The rationale is no different from that outlined for other fractures, but in the case of the pelvis it is more urgent.

In units experienced in dealing with this type of injury the placement of an external fixator on the pelvis may be part of the "C" component of the initial resuscitation and stabilisation of the patient. There may, however, be a serious conflict of interest if an abdominal injury is suspected, and unless the surgical teams have learned to work closely together the patient may die. A fixator may be applied within 5–10 minutes, if necessary in the emergency department, and it should be done before the abdomen is opened. It need not interfere with access to the abdomen, computed tomography, peritoneal lavage, or ultrasonography.

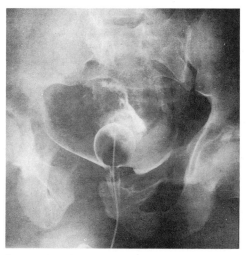

Cystogram of a bladder full of haematoma with extravasation of contrast due to a torn anterior bladder wall.

Damage to pelvic organs

Damage to pelvic organs is common, particularly to the urinary tract. If such damage is suspected (because of blood in the external meatus, perineal haematoma, or displacement of the prostate on rectal examination) urethral catheterisation should not be attempted. Instead an urgent retrograde urethrogram should be done; if injury is ruled out a catheter can be passed but if injury is confirmed an urgent urological opinion should be sought.

Damage to abdominal organs

Abdominal examination may be equivocal if there is a major pelvic injury. Peritoneal lavage can be done but the clinician should be cautious about interpreting the result. If the returned fluid is not frank blood the red cell count in the fluid should be measured (*see* Chapter 9). Opening the abdomen without good reason could do more harm than good. The problem is that blood may enter the peritoneal cavity from the retroperitoneal haematoma associated with a pelvic fracture so the result could be positive without damage to other organs. A negative result indicates no necessity for a laparotomy but a positive result does not always mean that there are other sources of bleeding. Ultrasound and computed tomography may help to make the diagnosis of solid organ injury, and assess the amount of blood free in the peritoneal cavity. Continuous monitoring of the haemoglobin concentration is essential because the blood loss may be immense.

Disruption of the pelvic ring with extensive damage to the pelvic blood vessels is an important cause of death in multiple trauma. Close cooperation between orthopaedic and general surgeons is critical to avoid unnecessary deaths, and it is unlikely that harm will be done by applying an external fixator to help stabilise the patient haemodynamically.

Radiology

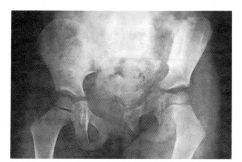

Vertical shear disruption of left hemipelvis.

Only when the multiply injured patient is resuscitated and stable and the three essential radiographs—of the chest, lateral cervical spine, and pelvis—have been performed should radiographs of limbs be considered. The standard two projections at right angles to one another are appropriate and must include the whole bone suspected of being fractured and the adjacent joints. Radiographs must be scrutinised for joint dislocations and subluxations that may be associated with fractures. Beware of requesting extensive radiographic studies if this requires the patient to be moved from the resuscitation area and its monitoring facilities.

Splintage

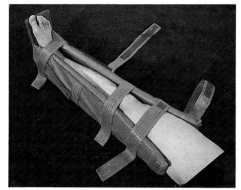

Leg splint.

The correct use of splintage will afford considerable pain relief, avert further soft tissue damage, and facilitate transport. To be effective the splint must immobilise the joint above and below the fracture and include the bone on either side of a dislocation. The arm is best supported by a simple sling and bandaged to the body. The forearm and wrist are immobilised on padded splints or pillows. The hand should be splinted in a functional position—that is, gripping a bandage roll. Femoral shaft fractures may be adequately controlled only by using fixed traction splints such as the Thomas splint or the modern equivalent. A traction force is applied to the leg or foot and is countered by a proximal pelvic bar. Low pressure (30 mmHg) inflatable double walled polyvinyl jacket splints are now commonly used to immobilise tibial, ankle, and forearm fractures—they are easy to use and effective.

Compartment syndromes

Multiply injured patients with reduced tissue perfusion and oxygenation are at high risk of developing compartment syndromes. Increasing swelling in the unyielding fascial compartments, particularly in the forearm and lower leg, as a result of tissue contusion, bleeding, or ischaemia may result in autoinfarction of the compartment muscle. The clinical symptoms and signs are increasing pain, sensory deficit in the distribution of the peripheral nerves passing through that compartment, progressive swelling and tension, and pain on passive muscle stretching. The presence of peripheral pulses does not exclude an evolving compartment syndrome.

If signs of a compartment syndrome develop all potentially constricting dressings, casts, and splints should be released. If rapid recovery is not observed then prompt fasciotomy should be performed. A high index of suspicion must be maintained in the unconscious patient and continuous instrumented compartment pressure monitoring may be indicated. Compartment pressures of greater than 30 mmHg are considered abnormal. It is a fallacy that compartment syndromes do not develop in patients with open fractures—an incidence of 15% has been reported.

Traumatic amputations

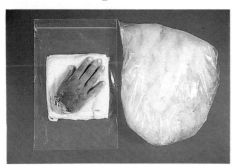

Amputation is a catastrophic life threatening injury. Haemorrhage must be controlled as a priority. Replantation is possible in certain instances. In these cases the amputated part should be cleaned; wrapped in a sterile cloth that has been soaked in saline; and sealed in a sterile plastic bag, which is then immersed in a container of crushed ice and water. The limb must not be allowed to freeze. Rapid transfer to the definitive care centre is essential. Amputated parts that are unsuitable for replantation may be a source of bone, skin, vessel, and nerve grafts and should not be discarded.

Management of an amputated hand.

Definitive management of fractures

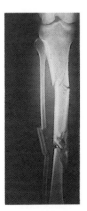
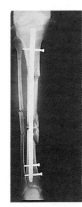

Internally fixed fractured tibia.

Closed fractures

The option of either surgical or conservative treatment of closed fractures available in patients with an isolated limb injury is inappropriate in the multiply injured patient. The incidence of, and the morbidity and mortality associated with, the adult respiratory distress syndrome, fat embolism, and late systemic sepsis are considerably reduced if the major long bone fractures are stabilised by internal or external fixation within 24 hours. This also results in easier nursing of the patient and a reduction in requirements for narcotic analgesia.

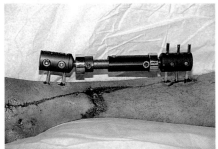

Externally fixed fracture.

Open fractures

The soft tissue damage and the risk of infection are the two critical factors determining outcome in patients with serious open fractures of the limbs. The treatment employed in the first few hours can determine the difference between complete recovery and lifelong disability. In remembering that the infecting organisms are the contaminating organisms, samples for culture should be obtained at the outset. The priorities are to reduce the size of the infecting inoculum by physical cleaning and to ensure that all devitalized tissue is excised.

In a multiply injured patient with a reduced oxygen delivery and an anticipated rise in tissue pressure, wound hypoxia and an increased susceptibility to infection are inevitable. Closure of the wound is therefore rarely indicated.

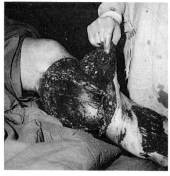

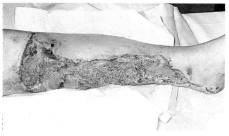

Soft tissue damage to the leg after a degloving injury (top); late flap necrosis was treated by excision and application of the split skin graft (meshed) obtained at the first operation (bottom).

Toilet of the wound is often performed inadequately. The surrounding skin should be shaved and particulate debris removed by scrubbing the wound with a brush. Meticulous exploration of the wound is necessary, and all recesses should be liberally irrigated by using a squirt and suck technique. Large volumes of warm saline or antiseptic solution are necessary (4–10 litres). Pressurised pulsed irrigation systems are now commercially available.

The wound is extended to facilitate examination as required. All non-viable muscle, fascia, and fat is carefully but radically excised. Fasciotomies may be performed once the wound has been thoroughly cleaned. Skin flaps of dubious viability are best dealt with by taking a split skin graft from the flap surface. This will serve to delineate the margin of viability, (the dead area will show no capillary bleeding). The harvested graft may be reapplied later if necrosis of the flap occurs. Small loose fragments of bone should be removed. Occasionally, large mechanically important fragments may be retained to help fracture fixation.

Most open fractures are unstable. Stabilisation is now recognised to promote tissue healing. A variety of methods are employed; the application of an external skeletal fixator is currently the most popular; this facilitates wound access and nursing care. Closure of the skin defect within seven days with a split skin graft, myocutaneous flap, or microvascular free flap as appropriate will appreciably reduce the risk of infection and rate of non-union of these fractures.

Conclusions

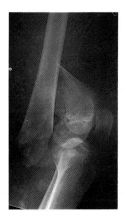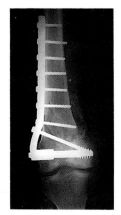

Unstable displaced supracondylar fracture of the femur (left); after internal fixation (right).

The assessment and management of limb trauma should always be secondary to resuscitation and management of life threatening conditions. A knowledge of the mechanism of injury and careful examination are essential if all of the sustained injuries are to be identified. Assessment of the peripheral circulation is crucial to allow early detection and management of potentially limb threatening injuries. Appropriate reduction of fractures and dislocations combined with correct splintage will reduce pain and can prevent serious complications.

A high level of suspicion is necessary in the multiply injured patient to identify nerve injuries and detect evolving compartment syndromes. Frequent reassessment and recordings of the circulation and neurological function of an injured limb are essential. The seriousness of open fracture wounds should be appreciated and an aggressive approach to wound toilet adopted. Urgent operative fixation of the major fractures within the first 24 hours will contribute to a reduction in mortality and morbidity.

The illustrations of leg trauma were reproduced by kind permission of Mr A Cobb, Mr I Hudson, and Mr R Birch, and the radiograph of the pelvic fracture by Dr D Stoker. The pictures of the leg splint and amputated hand were taken by the department of medical photography, Royal National Orthopaedic Hospital, London.

12 MEDICAL PROBLEMS

T D Wardle, Peter Driscoll

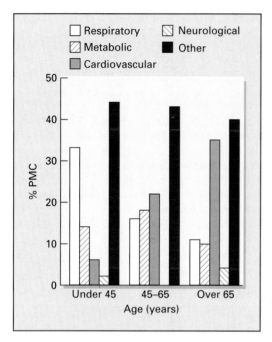

Graph showing how the incidence and type of premorbid condition (PMC) varies with age in UK trauma victims.

This chapter concentrates on health before injury and how it can influence both the clinical picture and the response to resuscitation. Management of these coexisting medical problems during the resuscitation phase will also be discussed.

Prevalence and effect

Only recently has attention been focused on the incidence, type, and effect of premorbid conditions on the outcome of a trauma patient. In the United States, their incidence ranges from 4.8% to 16%. This is dwarfed by the United Kingdom, where such conditions occur in 39% of major trauma patients. Despite these geographic differences, all studies have shown that there is an increase in the mortality rate of trauma victims with premorbid conditions. Furthermore, they are found in all age groups but, not surprisingly, their frequency increases with age.

Assessment and management

Conditions that compromise the airway

- Pseudobulbar palsy
- Bulbar palsy
- Macroglossia
- Progressive systemic sclerosis

The presence of premorbid conditions must not deflect the clinician from the ABCDE approach to the trauma patient. Instead, the medical problems at each stage in this process should be considered.

Airway and cervical spine immobilisation

Airway—Several medical conditions may compromise the airway (see box). Although these can influence airway management with simple adjuncts, they do not usually cause problems with endotracheal intubation. In contrast, difficulties may arise if the temperomandibular joints are affected by rheumatoid arthritis. In severe cases it may be impossible to open the mouth wide enough to allow oral intubation. Consequently other methods of securing the airway should be considered (see chapter 3), taking into account the urgency of the situation.

Immobilisation of cervical spine—Patients with rheumatoid disease or ankylosing spondylitis may have spinal involvement with the potential for rigidity, instability, and hence cervical cord injury. Furthermore, the amount of force required to cause injury can be quite small. Care should therefore be taken when clearing and securing the airway. In both conditions it is safer to assume that a cervical spine injury is present and maintain in-line immobilisation until it can be excluded clinically and radiologically.

Breathing

Respiratory diseases are common and many trauma victims present with coexisting pulmonary pathology. This can lead to diagnostic problems, especially when the patient has sustained a chest injury. Several respiratory conditions may not be apparent on initial assessment but clues can be gained from the history, examination, treatment response, arterial blood gas results, and chest radiograph. Arterial blood gas results are invaluable but must be interpreted in the light of the clinical situation. For example, hypoxia in an adequately ventilated

Progressive systemic sclerosis.

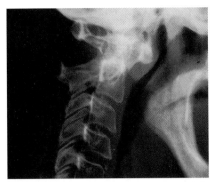

Rheumatoid cervical spine—atlantoaxial subluxation.

> **The presence of chronic pulmonary disease in trauma patients should be regarded as an early indication for ventilation**

Causes of pulmonary oedema

- Ischaemic heart disease
- Valvular disease
- Inhalation of noxious substances
- Pulmonary parenchymal injury
- Adult respiratory distress syndrome
- Neurological injury
- Myocardial trauma

Clinical features of fat emboli

- Tachypnoea
- Petechial rash
- Neurological signs

Premorbid conditions causing pulmonary emboli

- Stasis—for example, sitting during a long journey
- Cardiovascular
- Metabolic
- Malignancy
- Locomotor
- Haematological
- Others—for example, sepsis, dehydration

patient indicates that there could be underlying pulmonary emboli, sepsis, or contusion. In contrast, metabolic acidosis in trauma victims, especially when associated with an increased anion gap, usually indicates that there is hypoperfusion resulting in lactic acidosis.

Chronic bronchitis and emphysema—These are common in injured patients. Due to the deleterious effect of hypoxia following trauma, these patients require a fractional inspired oxygen of at least 0.85% irrespective of whether they have a hypoxic drive or not. Subsequently the oxygen concentration can be adjusted according to arterial blood gas results.

Bronchospasm—An AMPLE history will help determine if this is due to inhalation of noxious compounds or coexisting asthma. In both cases, bronchodilators should be given, with hydrocortisone added according to the clinical situation. It is also important to remember that asthmatic patients have an increased risk of developing a pneumothorax, especially if they require positive ventilation.

Pulmonary oedema—This can result from many causes but is usually a sequel to ischaemic heart disease and to a lesser extent mitral/aortic valve disease. This is particularly true if it is already present when the patient arrives in the accident and emergency department (providing their transfer has not been delayed). These patients will benefit from early endotracheal intubation, ventilation, and measurement of right and left heart pressures. Only in this way can the correct fluid resuscitation be achieved.

Pleural effusions—Many medical conditions, including left ventricular failure, pleuropulmonary malignancy, rheumatoid disease, and progressive systemic sclerosis may present with pleural effusions. Even if they are known to exist, a chest drain is still the management of choice. This not only reduces pulmonary embarrassment but also ensures that coexisting trauma is not present.

Pulmonary emboli—Following skeletal injury, in particular multiple fractures, fat emboli may result. While pulmonary signs predominate a variety of other clinical signs may be present. Irrespective of the many potential causes of massive pulmonary embolism, it usually presents as electromechanical dissociation. As thrombolysis would be precluded in the presence of multiple injuries, management is symptomatic and oxygen should be administered immediately.

Circulation and haemorrhage control

Hypotension

A low blood pressure following major trauma is usually due to hypovolaemia. However, if the patient fails to respond to fluid administration and there is no evidence of any occult bleed, then consider an underlying medical condition. As a minimum the clinician will require a:

- Full history and physical examination
- 12 lead ECG
- Full blood count
- Urea, glucose, and electrolyte analysis
- Arterial blood gas analysis
- Chest radiograph.

The presence of distended neck veins may indicate cardiac tamponade, pulmonary embolus, or right ventricular failure (from whatever cause). Further investigation will be required to determine the precise diagnosis.

Occult blood loss may occur in the gastrointestinal tract secondary to trauma. It may, however, reflect pre-existent peptic ulcer disease or inflammation. These may be exacerbated by stress ulceration, in particular related to burns (Curling's ulcers) or neurological injury (Cushing's ulcers).

Trauma victims presenting in *septic shock* are unusual unless there has been a prolonged delay in extrication or transfer. These patients may have hypotension initially, but they also have warm, well perfused peripheries. This is a useful physical sign in the differential diagnosis of hypotension.

Medical problems

Premorbid conditions that give rise to hypotension

Pulmonary:
  Embolism
  Tension pneumothorax
  Severe bronchospasm

Hypovolaemia:
  Diuretic
  Gastrointestinal bleed
  Adrenal insufficiency

Cardiac:
  Left/right ventricular failure
  Dysrhythmia
  Cardiac tamponade
  Pericardial effusion
  Septicaemia
  Uraemia
  Opiates

Circulatory:
  Diuretic
  Vasodilators
  Septicaemia
  Spinal cord injury
  Anaphylaxis
  Autonomic dysfunction

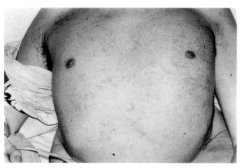

Petechial rash secondary to fat emboli.

Blind treatment of patients with diuretics or vasodilators may precipitate or exacerbate tissue hypoxia

Potential problems caused by pacemakers

- Damage to pacemaker/wire
- Pacemaker failure
- Inappropriate function
- Mask myocardial damage or bradycardia
- Inappropriate response to fluid resuscitation (especially if the pacemaker has a fixed rate)

Hypotension is an important sequal to adrenal and, rarely, pituitary insufficiency. The chances of it occurring in trauma victims are increasing because glucocorticoids are used in a variety of conditions. Consequently these patients may have suboptimal adrenal function, even if the steroid dose has been withdrawn gradually. In such circumstances any acute stress, including trauma, can precipitate an Addisonian crisis. This may be manifested by hypotension unresponsive to treatment or following stabilisation, recurrent hypotension, vomiting, confusion, or even coma. Be aware that the classic electrolyte changes are not always present.

If an Addisonian crisis is suspected then the patient should be given 300 mg of hydrocortisone intravenously. This should be repeated daily until it is convenient to perform a short synacthen test. Some indication as to the presence of the disease may be gained from a random serum cortisol concentration, which should be taken before hydrocortisone is administered.

Patients with left ventricular failure, uraemia, progressive systemic sclerosis, or rheumatoid disease may already have a pericardial effusion before the injury. If there is clinical evidence of a pericardial effusion then pericardiocentesis should be performed, not only to improve cardiac function but also to exclude associated pericardial or myocardial trauma.

Hypertension—This is always a concern. The history and physical examination are important, enabling the differentiation between acute and chronic hypertension. Acute hypertension may reflect increased intracranial pressure but other circulatory signs are usually present, in particular bradycardia. Persistent or fluctuating hypertension can indicate the presence of phaeochromocytoma. While this is a rare condition it does present problems for the unwary. Patients with acute hypertension need invasive monitoring and the intravenous administration of both α and β blockers so that a careful controlled reduction of blood pressure can be achieved.

Ischaemic heart disease—This is the most prevalent disease in the Western world and if present will be exacerbated by blood loss, hypoxia, hypovolaemia, or hypotension. If the patient is unconscious, however, myocardial infarction may not be apparent. In these cases a 12 lead ECG and cardiac monitoring are essential. Hypotension is a particularly difficult problem in patients with ischaemic heart disease and haemorrhage. The commonest cause is blood loss, but this may not be the only one because it may be the product of blood loss and heart failure. It is therefore crucial that fluid replacement should be governed by accurate invasive monitoring.

Arrhythmias—These may be a reflection of underlying myocardial ischaemia. However, there are other causes—in particular, hypoxia, electrolyte disturbance, increased intracranial pressure, and coexistent drug therapy. Arrhythmias may in turn precipitate or exacerbate hypotension, cardiac failure, hypoxia, and loss of consciousness. Tachydysrhythmias can be treated with drugs if the patient is haemodynamically stable with no evidence of cardiac failure or impaired consciousness. As all these drugs depress myocardial function, a tachydysrhythmia in the presence of cardiac failure should be treated with appropriate cardioversion.

Valvar disease—Aortic valve disease is on the increase, especially in the elderly population. The pulse pressure which can result may be misdiagnosed as an early indicator of shock. Excessive fluid administration in this situation can result in left, or biventricular failure. Cardiac decompensation may also occur because of underlying ischaemic heart disease or myocardial contusion. Patients should be given prophylactic antibiotics as soon as it is convenient providing there are no contraindications. Ampicillin 1 g and gentamycin 80 mg repeated after 12 hours is standard practice.

Cardiac pacemakers—These can profoundly influence the clinical picture following major trauma (see box).

Chronic anaemia—This is a common condition. Unfortunately information as to the presence and type of anaemia may not be available from the initial haemoglobin estimation. Therefore patients should be transfused according to their haemodynamic parameters rather than their haemoglobin concentration. Haemoglobinopathies, in particular

Causes of chronic anaemia

- Chronic renal failure
- Chronic liver disease
- Acute intestinal inflammation
- Chronic intestinal inflammation
- Multi-system disease
- Haemolytic anaemia
- Post gastrectomy
- Ileal resection

Coagulation disorders

- Thrombocytopenia (especially if $< 20 \times 10^9/l$)
- Congenital coagulation defects—for example, haemophilia
- Acquired coagulation defects—for example, malabsorption
- Disseminated intravascular coagulation

It is mandatory that all trauma patients have a serum glucose estimation as hypoglycaemia is easy to treat but easy to miss!

Causes of fits and coma

Drugs/chemicals:
Cocaine, solvent abuse, tricyclic overdose, alcohol, lead poisoning

Infections:
Meningitis, encephalitis, toxoplasmosis, malaria, intracerebral abscess

Vascular:
Thromboembolic disease, hypertension, dysrhythmia

Metabolic:
Hypoglycaemia, hyperglycaemia, uraemia, electrolyte imbalance, hypocalcaemia, anoxia, hepatic encephalopathy

Intracerebral tumours

sickle-cell disease, may precipitate or be precipitated by major trauma. Furthermore, acute pain, in particular abdominal pain, may reflect a sickle crisis rather than intraperitoneal injury. Tenderness is not uncommon and under these circumstances diagnostic peritoneal lavage or computed tomography is recommended.

Coagulopathy—Whether this is due to a bleeding diathesis or a procoagulant disease, it can profoundly influence the patient's response to both trauma and resuscitation. If a history is not available and clinical features, in particular chronic liver disease, are not obvious, then this problem will only come to light during resuscitation. If there is any suspicion of coagulopathy then it is advisable to check both the activated partial thromboplastin and prothrombin times. These should be corrected appropriately.

Electrolyte imbalance—This is not uncommon, especially in patients taking diuretics. Hyperkalaemia is likely to be the most important electrolyte problem in the acute situation. This should not be ascribed to a haemolysed sample because patients can have coexisting renal dysfunction, metabolic acidosis in association with shock, diabetic ketoacidosis, or even tissue (especially muscular) necrosis. This is particularly important in patients who have chronic or acute renal failure where underperfusion may exacerbate the situation and warrant early consultation with a nephrologist.

Cardiac transplants—The type of transplant will govern whether the myocardium is able to respond either to direct neural, sympathetic stimulation or indirectly to circulating catecholamines.

Disability

With the increasing numbers of elderly patients there is a coexisting increase in cerebrovascular disease. It is important to remember that hypoglycaemia has many manifestations and may mimic a stroke.

Many neurological problems can be identified when assessing airway, breathing, and circulation. Fits or coma are usually ascribed to intracerebral injury, however, in the presence of a normal computed tomography scan other conditions need to be considered (see box). Hyponatraemia or hypocalcaemia may be precipitated by rapid volume expansion whereas hypernatraemia can be precipitated or exacerbated by dehydration and result in cerebral oedema (for example, in association with excessive burns).

Many of the chronic neurological diseases, stroke or demyelination may present with lateralising signs. These can mimic or mask occult intracerebral trauma. The presence of these signs necessitates computed tomography if no history is available.

Autonomic dysfunction may not only mask the patient's response to trauma and fluid resuscitation but can also mimic spinal cord injury. With the exception of diabetes mellitus most causes of autonomic dysfunction are rare. Ideally patients should be treated as though they have an acute spinal injury. Invasive monitoring and cautious fluid resuscitation are therefore mandatory and inotropic agents should be considered.

Malignant hyperpyrexia and the neuroleptic malignant syndrome are potentially fatal disorders that may not be evident during the primary survey and may only be diagnosed during or following anaesthesia. These conditions necessitate prompt treatment with dantrolene and measures to maintain an appropriate core temperature.

Exposure

Hypothermia can precipitate, or be the result of, major trauma. Appropriate means to correct the body temperature include the use of warmed intravenous fluids and overhead heating in the resuscitation room (see chapter 3).

Medical problems

AMPLE History

Many medical problems will be identified in trauma patients providing that an AMPLE history has been obtained. Information may have to be sought not only from the patient but also from the general practitioner, hospital records, relatives and witnesses.

Allergies—These are unlikely to influence the management of a trauma patient unless they either precipitated the trauma or resulted from drugs given. A range of clinical manifestations can occur. Anaphylactic shock, the most sinister manifestation, requires immediate intravenous adrenaline.

Medication—Many patients are taking medications and these may not be known at the time of resuscitation. β blockers, calcium channel antagonists, ACE inhibitors, and, to a lesser extent, nitrates are important because they modify the cardiovascular response to both trauma and resuscitation. The use of oral steroids is common and an Addisonian crisis can be precipitated if these drugs are omitted.

The use of recreational drugs may also precipitate or modify the patient's response to trauma. Alcohol influences presentation, treatment, and outcome of major trauma. The link between alcohol and road traffic accidents is well established.

Alcohol can produce a variety of clinical manifestations, as can its withdrawal. In the presence of chronic alcohol consumption adequate thiamine should be administered and careful control of withdrawal symptoms with chlordiazepoxide is mandatory.

Past medical history—This is extremely important as this will alert the physician to factors that may influence the clinical presentation or response to treatment.

Last meal—In addition to needing this information as part of the anaesthetic work up for surgery, it can also help explain the cause of hypoglycaemia in the trauma patient.

Environment—Information about the environment is important in explaining hypothermia. If a low core temperature cannot be attributed to exposure to the cold it should alert the physician to the presence of occult pathology, in particular pancreatitis, diabetes, hypothyroidism, and phenothiazine overdose.

AMPLE history

- **A** Allergies
- **M** Medication
- **P** Past medical history
- **L** Last meal
- **E** Event/environment

Summary

It is best to exclude disease rather than to ignore it

Medical problems occur frequently in trauma patients. Not only can they cause the incident but they may also result from the injury or its subsequent treatment. Depending on the type of condition, they can have a tremendous impact on the resuscitation and the patient's subsequent outcome.

To overcome these problems it is essential that the clinician keeps to the "ABCDE" system of trauma resuscitation and considers the potential medical problems if the patient fails to respond to treatment in the expected way. An AMPLE history is invaluable, especially when supplemented by information from the hospital notes and general practitioner.

It follows that the physician has an important role in the management of major trauma patients.

The illustrations were prepared by the department of medical illustration, Salford Royal Hospitals NHS trust. The photograph on p 66 is reproduced with the patient's permission.

13 RADIOLOGICAL ASSESSMENT

N M Perry, M D Lewars, Peter Driscoll

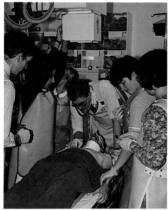

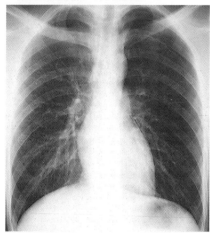

Left sided pneumothorax. The separated white line at the upper left heart border indicates pneumomediastinum.

The mainstay of radiological investigation of trauma in the resuscitation room is the plain radiograph, which is available in all accident and emergency departments. Many immediate management decisions can be made with the aid of such radiographs, which show possible causes of cardiorespiratory compromise and detail any major bone or soft tissue injury. The development of pneumothorax, haemothorax, or early signs of aortic rupture may be clearly shown. Radiological investigation should not interfere with the mechanics of resuscitation or be allowed to delay appropriate surgery.

The experienced radiographer is an invaluable member of the emergency team. He or she can advise on the effects that positioning and resuscitation procedures may have on the images produced and give guidance as to possible delays caused by various radiographic techniques.

Unnecessary exposure of the patient and, particularly, of members of staff to damaging ionising radiation must be avoided. Every radiograph should have a purpose. The quality of each image will depend on the time and effort taken to produce it. Full radiological evaluation may be deferred in patients with peripheral injuries that are not life threatening, particularly if there are other patients with trauma to be assessed.

Two important considerations in cases of major trauma are whether recognised focal injury has had hidden consequences and whether there is clinically occult damage that can be signalled early by radiography. For example, a rib or sternal fracture may be clinically quite apparent, but there may be an underlying haemopericardium; likewise a pneumothorax or pneumomediastinum may become apparent only on radiography.

Radiological survey

General principles of radiological assessment

- Follow the ABCs system of interpretation
- Plain films are most useful in the resuscitation room
- Imaging must not interfere with resuscitation
- All patients with major trauma should have the following radiographs taken
  —Cervical spine (lateral)
  —Chest
  —Pelvis
- Two views are needed to exclude bone injury
- If in doubt seek radiological advice

Patients with major trauma should have immediate lateral cervical spine, chest, and pelvic radiographs taken, usually at the end of the primary survey or during the secondary survey. The images should be assessed using the "ABCs" system as soon as they are processed and serve as a baseline for future comparison.

The patient is usually supine and immobilised by a variety of intravenous lines, and airway devices and by a stabilising cervical collar. These factors modify the quality of the radiographs. Some areas of the film may be overexposed (dark), necessitating the use of a bright light. Major trauma may affect different organ systems and parts of the body simultaneously. Once an abnormality has been identified and evaluated as far as possible attention should be turned to the possibility of an additional serious injury.

Fractures are usually represented by lucent (dark) lines, which may or may not cross the entire bone. Occasionally, overlapping fragments may result in a linear density (white line) rather than lucency. Sometimes the only sign of fracture may be the alteration of the internal trabecular pattern.

Radiological assessment

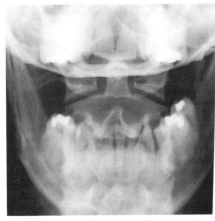

Supplementary "open mouth" odontoid peg radiograph showing symmetry of the lateral masses of C1 with regard to the peg and body of C2.

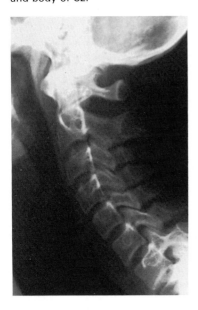

Two radiographs taken from different angles are required to assess any fractured bone: a single view rarely excludes a fracture. The bone contours should be inspected for irregular steps. Abnormal angulation, particularly in children, should be regarded as suspicious. With few exceptions (one being the knee) joint surfaces should be parallel and congruent.

Injured joints usually lead to effusions, even without fracture. Effusions may be visualised as soft tissue densities in relation to the joint capsule or by displacement of fat planes. Local haemorrhage from a skeletal fracture is also visualised as a soft tissue density with displacement or effacement of fat planes.

Soft tissue injuries may be more important than fractures, even when the two are associated. An atypical or asymmetrical soft tissue density may represent a haematoma or other fluid collection. The presence of gas in the soft tissues, visualised as dark streaks or bubbles in the tissue planes, is a sign of compound or penetrating injury involving the bowel, lungs, or neck structures.

Many accident victims have had previous trauma or disease—for example, degenerative change in the cervical spine—which will be apparent in the radiograph. Age related osteopenia predisposes patients to fractures, especially vertebral wedge compression fractures. The age of fractures may be estimated from their density, cortical thickness, and trabecular continuity. In patients with major trauma it is safest to assume that all fractures are new. Familiarity with the variety of normal appearances can develop only with experience.

Finally, if there is any doubt or mismatch of clinical and radiological appearances ask a radiologist for advice. Recent air, rail, and boating disasters have shown the advantage of experienced radiologists being present in the accident department: they are able to provide early authoritative interpretations of radiographs, direct the taking of further films, perform any necessary further investigation, and redistribute imaging services to accommodate the volume of work.

ABCs system of radiographic interpretation

A—**A**lignment and **A**dequacy
B—**B**ones
C—**C**artilage/joints
S—**S**oft tissues

Cervical spine

Adequacy	All seven vertebrae shown
	Enough lateral projection for assessment
Alignment	Check the spinolaminar/marginal/interspinous lines
	Check the anteroposterior depth of the spinal canal
Bones	Study each individual vertebra
	Ensure there are no bony fragments
	Look for cortical continuity and obvious fracture lines
Cartilage/joints	Check disc spaces and facet joints
	Check predental space
Soft tissues	Look for local or generalised prevertebral swelling

Any multiply injured patient must be considered to have a cervical injury until proved otherwise. Manipulation or unguarded movement of the inadequately immobilised neck can cause cord damage, most commonly in patients with injuries below C3. It is important to realise that a lateral radiograph shows only 70%–90% of the important cervical injuries. It is therefore essential that this radiograph is supplemented by anterior, odontoid peg, and oblique views if there are clinical or radiological signs of cervical injury or any specific history. As these are best carried out in the radiology department, they cannot be performed until the patient is haemodynamically stable. Until this occurs the trauma victim's neck must remain immobilised.

Adequacy and alignment

Important cervical injury is associated with neurological damage in 40%–50% of cases; instability increases this risk by 10%–20%. Vital considerations are whether the radiological view supplied is adequate for assessment and whether there is evidence of either injury or instability.

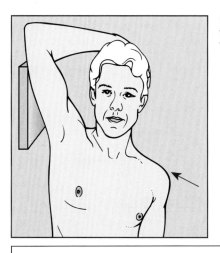

Position of patient for swimmer's view.

Important measurements

- Overriding of vertebral bodies:
  Without fracture—25% indicates unifacetal dislocation;
  50% indicates bifacetal dislocation
  With fracture—>3.5 mm indicates instability

- Depth of spinal canal—>13 mm

- Predental space—≤3 mm (adult)
  ≤5 mm (child)

- Depth of prevertebral soft tissue:
  Above larynx—≤7 mm
  Below larynx—≤22 mm (or depth of vertebral body)

Signs of cervical instability

- Angulation between vertebrae >10°
- Vertebral override >3.5 mm with fracture
- Complete facet override
- Facetal joint widening
- Interspinous "fanning"
- Vertebral body compression >25%

Classification of cervical injury

Stable injuries
- Hyperflexion—compression fracture (if <25%)
- Spinous process fracture
- Unifacetal dislocation
- Pure C1 arch fracture
- Pillar fracture
- Lower cervical burst fracture

Unstable injuries
- Hyperflexion "teardrop" injury
- Hyperextension "teardrop" injury
- Traumatic spondylolisthesis of C2 (Hangman's fracture)
- Bilateral facet dislocation
- C2 posterior arch fracture
- Hyperextension fracture dislocation
- Jefferson fracture of C1
- Basal peg fracture

All seven cervical vertebrae as well as the C7-T1 junction must be visualised in the lateral radiograph. Injuries often occur at C6/7, with C1/2 next in frequency. The "swimmer's" view of the cervicothoracic junction is helpful when the lower cervical spine has not been fully visualised (see chapter 8) but is difficult to interpret and is unsafe if cervicothoracic injury is strongly suspected as it requires manipulation of the patient. Anteroposterior oblique views with tube angulation of 30° will show the lower cervical spine and also the facet joints and foraminae. The patient need not be moved for these views.

Alignment of the cervical spine radiograph is assessed by the following lines. Each line should be smooth with no angulation.

Anterior and posterior marginal lines connect the surfaces of adjacent vertical bodies and represent the sites of the longitudinal ligaments.

The spinolaminar line connects the white lines where laminae of each vertebra meet to form the spinous processes. C2 is frequently posterior to this line by up to 3 mm in normal subjects.

Spinous processes should be roughly equidistant and converge to a point behind the patient's neck. They should not diverge or "fan out".

Vertebral canal—The anteroposterior diameter of the vertebral canal, measured between the spinolaminar and posterior marginal lines, is of prime importance at the site of cervical expansion of the cord—between C3 and C6. If it is <13 mm, particularly in the presence of bone injury, the cord is at risk or already damaged. Note any pre-existing degenerative cervical spine changes with osteophytes in elderly patients; cord damage can occur in these patients without noticeable narrowing. Likewise, spinal stenosis may be a longstanding feature due to posterior osteophytes.

Soft tissues—Above the level of the laryngeal inlet the prevertebral soft tissue should have a thickness of ≤7 mm. There should be no localised swelling. Below the larynx the tracheal air shadow should not be separated from the anterior marginal line by no more than the equivalent of the anteroposterior diameter of a vertebral body: an upper limit of 22 mm is often quoted. Again there should be no localised swelling. Tracheal deviation in the anteroposterior view may be important providing there is no goitre present. Presphenoidal adenoidal enlargement in children and young adults may simulate a mass anterior to C1/2. Neck flexion and crying may also increase the depth of the prevertebral soft tissues substantially.

Bones

Cartilage and joints—Vertebral bodies should be inspected for evidence of fracture. The height of each vertebral body should be similar anteriorly and posteriorly. A difference in height of >2 mm between the front and back is important and may indicate a crush fracture. Fractures of the spinous processes are usually shown in the lateral view; fractures of the posterior arch, however, may be apparent only in oblique projections.

The space between the anterior cortex of the odontoid peg and the posterior cortex of the anterior arch of the atlas (the predental space) should be ≤3 mm in an adult (≤5 mm in a child). Greater distances imply atlantoaxial instability.

Disc spaces should be roughly equal in height unless there are associated degenerative changes. The height of any disc space should be even throughout. Angulation of >10° between apposed vertebral body end plates implies instability of traumatic origin.

A forward slip of one vertebral body on its neighbour may indicate dislocation. Shift of up to 25% of the anteroposterior diameter of the body is seen with subluxation and with unilateral facet dislocation. Displacement of >50% is a sign of probable bilateral facet joint dislocation. A forward slip of one vertebral body on its neighbour of >3.5 mm in the presence of a fracture indicates an unstable fracture dislocation.

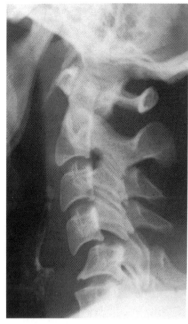

Forward slip of C4 on C5 of >50%. No fracture is present and the facets are overriding, indicating a bilateral facet dislocation.

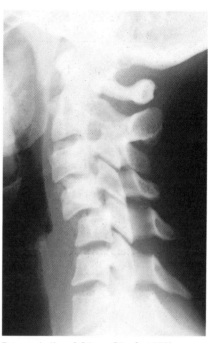

Forward slip of C4 on C5 of <25%. No fracture is visible. The disc space is slightly narrowed.

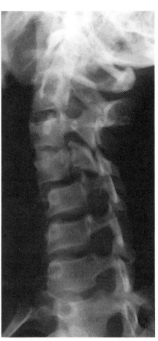

Supplementary oblique projection shows malalignment of the facet joints, indicating a unilateral facet dislocation.

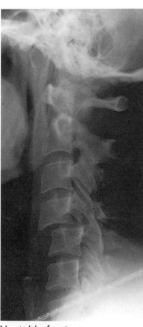

Unstable fracture subluxation. C4 has slipped forward on C5, the disc space is narrowed, and there is a fracture of the posterior elements and a fracture of the spinous process of C6.

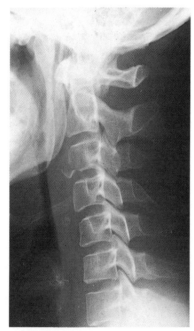

Hyperextension "teardrop" fracture of C3 showing avulsed anteroinferior fragment from the body of C3 and some localised prevertebral soft tissue swelling. This injury was unstable.

The two major mechanisms of cervical spine injury are hyperflexion and hyperextension. Hyperflexion is the commoner, causing 50%–80% of cervical spine injuries. There is a tendency for the posterior elements to be disrupted. Hyperextension injuries conversely tend to disrupt the anterior supports. "Teardrop" avulsion or compression fragments of the anterior aspect of a vertebral body may be the only residual features of major disruption and ensuing instability.

Compression fractures are generally stable. The Jefferson burst fracture of C1, however, is not, and the lateral radiograph may well show only soft tissue swelling. An open mouth view is essential to judge the integrity of C1 and the symmetry of its position on either side of the odontoid peg (see chapter 8). C2 fractures may be associated. Neurological damage is rare as the canal is wide at this level. Conversely, neurological damage caused by stable lower cervical compression fractures is fairly common due to posterior displacement of fragments into a relatively narrow canal. A wedge fracture in an elderly patient with osteopenia should be differentiated if possible as it is unlikely to be important.

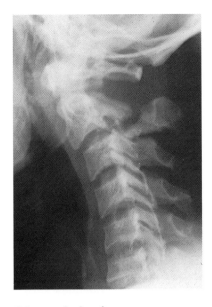
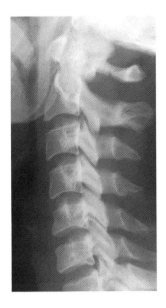

(Far left) "Hangman's" traumatic spondylolisthesis of C2. C2 is subluxed forward on C3 and the posterior elements are clearly separated. The posterior arch of C1 is also fractured. (Left) Pure C1 arch fracture. There is an undisplaced fracture line passing vertically through the posterior arch of C1. This injury was stable.

Fractures of the odontoid peg are commonest at its base. They are unstable, though neurological damage is uncommon. There is variable displacement, and soft tissue swelling is often seen only in the lateral radiograph. Ideally, a fractured peg should be excluded before intubation is attempted. An experienced anaesthetist may, however, be willing to proceed without radiological proof if the clinical situation dictates.

Chest injuries

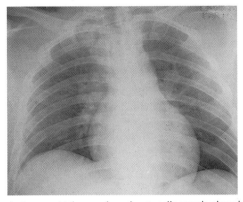

Anteroposterior supine chest radiograph showing poor inspiration and prominent upper lobe vasculature.

About 25% of deaths caused by major trauma are due to thoracic damage. The most useful radiograph in patients with thoracic trauma is the erect posteroanterior view. In the resuscitation room, however, the standard radiograph is often the supine anteroposterior view, which has the disadvantage of causing apparent enlargement of heart and mediastinal shadows, distending the upper lobe vessels, and making inspiration less efficient. In the supine position pleural air collects anteroinferiorly, outlining the diaphragm and heart, while pleural fluid layers posteriorly giving ill defined opacification of the hemithorax.

Adequacy	Check for adequacy of inspiration, penetration of film, and artefacts of resuscitation
Alignment	Check natural curve of ribs and thoracic cage
	Check position of spinous processes with respect to medial ends of clavicles
Bones	Look for fracture lines and cortical continuity
	Rib fractures: How many ribs fractured? How many fractures/rib?
Cartilage/joints	Look particularly at the sternoclavicular joint
Soft tissues	Localised opacities may be pulmonary, pleural, artefactual, or chest wall
	Ensure density of each hemithorax is equal and mediastinum central
	Check smooth contour of diaphragm
	Observe the mediastinal outline and width
	Check aortic knuckle for contour and definition
	Look for abnormal gas in pleural, mediastinal, subcutaneous, and subphrenic spaces

Adequacy and alignment

Poor inspiration as well as rotation of the patient in relation to the radiographic beam may result in artefactually abnormal appearances. Ideally, five anterior ribs and ten posterior ribs should be counted above the level of the hemidiaphragm. The medial ends of the clavicles should be equidistant from the vertebral spinous processes.

The basic rules for assessment of the chest radiograph are that the transverse diameter of the heart should not be greater than half the transverse diameter of the thorax and that two thirds of the heart should lie to the left of the midline. Vascular distribution should be symmetrical on each side, and each hemithorax should have equal translucency. The hilar shadows should be clearly defined, with the left hilum being about 1–2 cm higher than the right. Cardiac, mediastinal, and diaphragmatic contours should be clearly outlined.

Radiological assessment

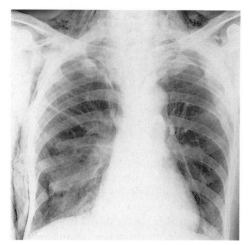

Extreme surgical emphysema and pneumomediastinum caused by multiple rib fractures. There is outlining of the pectoral muscle fibres on the right side.

Bones

All the bones visible on the chest radiograph must be assessed for breaks in the cortical margin or disruption of the trabecular pattern.

Injuries of the chest wall frequently accompany pelvic trauma. The fifth to ninth ribs are most commonly injured. Lower rib fractures may be associated with splenic, hepatic, or renal damage, while fractures of the first two ribs imply that the patient has sustained a considerable force and is likely to have associated cranial, cervical, or intrathoracic injury. A fracture of the first rib with displaced fragments carries a 60% risk of underlying major vascular damage. The presence of surgical emphysema in the neck or mediastinum in addition highlights the severity of the injury.

Flail chest occurs when multiple and adjacent rib fractures allow an area of the chest wall to move paradoxically with respiration. Sternal fractures are best shown in the lateral radiograph and may be associated with underlying pulmonary or cardiac injury. Complications caused by rib fractures include pneumothorax, haemothorax, and pulmonary contusion or laceration.

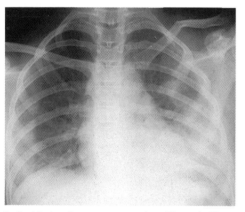

Left sided pulmonary contusion. There is ill defined opacification over the left mid-zone and base. Although the left clavicle is fractured, no obvious rib fracture is shown.

Cartilage and joints

All joints visible on the radiograph must be checked for congruity of the articular surfaces. Posterior sternoclavicular joint dislocation can be identified by obvious asymmetry at the manubrium, and there is associated risk of brachiocephalic vein disruption.

Soft tissue

Pulmonary and pleural features of injury—Sequelae of thoracic trauma include segmental, lobar, or pulmonary collapse. Features of opacification and alteration of hilar and fissure positions must be sought. Fluid aspiration causes patchy air space consolidation, typically in the upper lobes or apices of the lower lobe. Acute pulmonary oedema may appear solely as "bat's wing shadowing" extending from the hila resulting from fluid exudation into the alveolar spaces. Interstitial oedema is hallmarked by peribronchial thickening, the septal lines of interlobular fluid, and, indeed, pleural fluid. A pleural effusion may also indicate an abdominal injury such as splenic or hepatic laceration, and signs of subdiaphragmatic air from a visceral perforation should be sought in the upright chest radiograph.

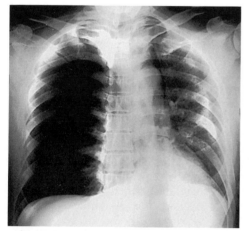

Right sided tension pneumothorax. The right hemithorax is very translucent with absent lung markings. There is flattening of the right dome of the diaphragm and considerable shift of the heart and mediastinum to the left.

Diaphragmatic injury—Rupture of the diaphragm is commoner on the left side and can be caused by either blunt or penetrating trauma. Haemothorax, pulmonary collapse due to compression, rib fractures, and hepatic or splenic injuries may coexist. Ruptures due to blunt trauma are usually larger and more immediately apparent. The appearances are easily misinterpreted as a subpulmonic effusion, loculated haemopneumothorax, or just a high hemidiaphragm of unknown cause. A contrast examination may be necessary to show bowel loops within the thorax.

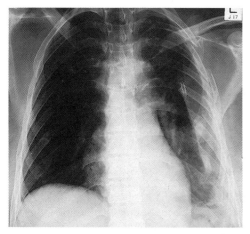

Flail chest caused by at least six fractured ribs both in the posterior axillary line as well as anteriorly.

Radiological signs of major thoracic trauma
- Mediastinal widening
- Mediastinal shift
- Mediastinal emphysema
- Multiple rib fractures
- Fractured first or second ribs
- Pleural fluid
- Loss of aortic definition

Mediastinal injuries—Penetrating injuries may result in mediastinal or pericardial emphysema. The former is apparent in the radiograph as a white line that parallels the mediastinal border, particularly on the left side. Free mediastinal air may extend to the neck, where streaky air lucencies are readily visible in the soft tissue planes. The tracheobronchial tree and oesophagus may be injured in patients with blunt, penetrating, or deceleration trauma. Oesophageal rupture typically causes mediastinal emphysema with an accompanying left sided pleural effusion. Bronchial fracture may cause segmental or lobar collapse but can be very subtle radiologically.

Major vascular and cardiac injuries—Major vascular and cardiac injuries may be found in association with sternal or first rib fractures and in patients with injuries caused by deceleration forces. Patients with aortic rupture may well survive to reach the resuscitation room. Vital features include mediastinal widening, loss of definition of the aortic knuckle, deviation to the right of the trachea, and thickening of the apical pleura on the left side (see chapter 4).

Cardiac and pericardial trauma may cause haemopericardium with the risk of tamponade. The heart size will be increased, but classically described features of a globular appearance and notable clarity of cardiac outline due to reduced motion are unreliable.

Pelvic injuries

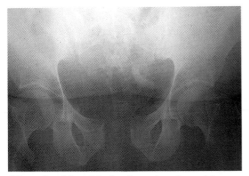

"Open book" pelvic fracture showing wide separation of the pubic symphysis and diastasis (widening) of the right sacroiliac joint.

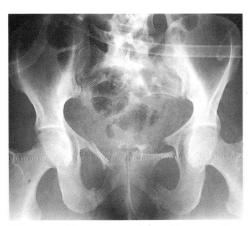

Bilateral pubic ramus fractures with separation (the "straddle" injury). Catheterisation for cystography has been performed. There is also an undisplaced left iliac wing fracture.

In 94% of cases a correct diagnosis can be made from just an anteroposterior radiograph of the pelvis. In the remaining 6% of cases, this radiograph needs to be supplemented by inlet, outlet and Judet (ie acetabular view at 45°) views. In addition, many patients with pelvic fractures require contrast examinations because of the high association of soft tissue damage. Computed tomography is also becoming an essential element in the preoperative work up of haemodynamically stable patients with pelvic trauma. Arteriography may be used diagnostically or for therapeutic embolisation of bleeding vessels.

As with the other radiographs described in this chapter, the antereoposterior view of the pelvis should be assessed using the "ABCs" system.

Adequacy and alignment

All the pelvis must be seen, including the iliac crests, hips and femurs distal to the lesser trochanters. Pelvic rotation is determined by lining up the symphysis pubis with the midline of the sacrum.

Radiological assessment

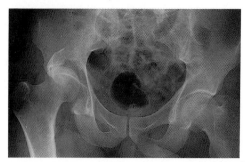

Acetabular fracture with posterior dislocation of the right femoral head. The acetabular fragment shows as a white line above the hip joint. The hip joint space is considerably widened medially and inferiorly.

Adequacy	Check that whole pelvis is visible and not too rotated
	Should include hips and necks of femurs
Alignment	Check smooth contours of the pelvic and obturator rings and Shenton's line
Bones	Look for cortical and trabecular interruption
	Ensure that there are no fragments or overlap
	Don't ignore the sacrum
Cartilage/joints	Check symmetry of hips and sacroiliac joints
	Check width of pubic symphysis
Soft tissues	Check fat and soft tissue planes both inside and outside the pelvis
	Look for abnormal gas shadows

Bones

The pelvic brim and the two obturator foramina should trace out smooth, uninterrupted circles. The superior aspect of the obturator fossa continues laterally along the inferior aspect of the femoral neck to form Shenton's line.

Disruption of these circles cannot occur at a single point. Therefore once one break is found a search must be made for a second fracture or joint diastasis. Significant opening of the sacroiliac joints is associated with tearing of the major blood vessels which overlie this joint. This radiological feature is therefore a sign of vascular damage and a potential source of major blood loss.

Fractures of the pelvic brim are caused by different types of forces. Lateral compression may result from inward rotation of the hemipelvis with disruption of the sacroiliac joint. The pubic rami are usually fractured and occasionally the sacrum as well. In contrast anteroposterior forces tend to drive the iliac wings apart and disrupt the symphysis (the "open book" fracture). Pubic ramus fractures may also be present and, when bilateral (the "straddle" injury), are associated with urethral damage. Vertical shear forces have the highest risk of producing vascular damage because they tend to displace the hemipelvis upwards in relation to the sacrum. Additional pelvic fractures will usually be present.

Individual fractures may also occur. Consequently the outer edges of the pelvis, as well as its internal trabecular pattern, should be assessed. The sacral foramina must also be assessed for symmetry. A break in their smooth border may be the only indicator of a lateral compression fracture.

Open fractures are important to detect because they are associated with a significant increase in mortality.

Cartilage and joints

All the joints must be assessed for congruity, disruption of the articular surfaces and widening.

The commonest type of acetabular fracture occurs in the posterior wall. It is accompanied by a posterior dislocation and is found in people who have sustained a strong anterior force to the femur whilst in the sitting position. A lateral force may result in a central dislocation with associated acetabular fracture. Nevertheless relocation, either spontaneously or by manipulation, may leave only subtle soft tissue changes. Anterior dislocation is rare.

Soft tissues

Intra and extrapelvic soft tissue planes must be assessed. Displacement by large haematomas may be the only indicator of fractures or vascular damage. Major pelvic trauma is associated with bladder rupture in 10%–15% of cases.

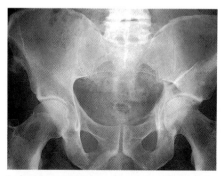

Left sided acetabular fracture with central dislocation of the femoral head. There is narrowing of the medial aspect of the hip joint space and medial displacement of the femoral head. Note the thick white line of overlapping bone fragments.

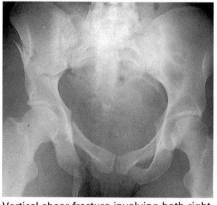

Vertical shear fracture involving both right sided pubic rami and iliac wing with a small amount of superior displacement. A sacral fracture is also visible.

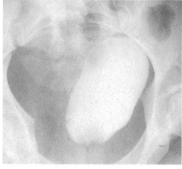

Contrast material within the bladder from an intravenous urogram shows bladder displacement by a large haematoma. The transverse sacral fracture can be clearly seen.

Skull injuries

Unnecessary importance is sometimes given to radiography of the skull. Criteria for its use have been proposed that essentially require that a neurological deficit of intracranial origin is present or that assessment of such a deficit is not possible. Once taken, this radiograph should be assessed using the "ABCs" system. Some features to aid differentiation of fractures from other lucencies appearing in the skull radiograph are given in the table.

Differentiation of lucencies in the skull

Feature	Artery	Vein	Suture	Fracture
Shape	Regular and roughly straight	Wandering	Tortuous but inner junction straight	Usually straight
Calibre	Even	Uneven	Even	Variable
Cortical margin	Present	Present	Present	Absent
Branching	Common, even	Common, irregular	Rare (for example, lambdoid suture)	May be stellate if depressed
Anatomical site	Fairly constant	Very variable	Constant	Anywhere

Adequacy	Ensure a good lateral view showing the vault, mandible and C1/2
Alignment	Check the contour of the skull tables and the relationship of the facial bones to the skull
Bones	Check for linear lucencies of fractures
	Do not ignore overlapping fragments causing white lines
Cartilage/joints	Look for obvious sutural diastasis and temporomandibular joint disruption
Soft tissues	Check for intracranial air
	Check for air or fluid levels in the sinuses
	Remember that the film may be "brow up"

Other imaging techniques

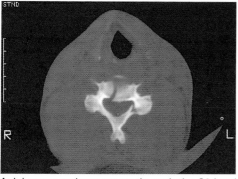

Axial computed tomogram through the C6 level shows not only the extent of the fracture through its body with some posterior fragment displacement but also a fracture through the arch (not apparent in the plain radiograph).

Ultrasonography may be used to assess damage to soft tissues, particularly in the abdomen. It can be used frequently in monitoring as it does not expose the patient to ionising radiation, though bowel gas and tenderness may preclude optimal imaging.

Computed tomography, angiography, and embolisation do not have a place in the resuscitation room, but they may alter the pattern of immediate management once the patient is clinically stable.

Computed tomography requires time for transfer and preparation of the patient, but this is repaid because minimum manipulation of the patient is necessary during investigation. The data obtained provide accurate assessment of the degree of internal damage as well as localising bone fragments and locating abnormal collections of air and fluid. The technique helps in determining the extent of spinal injury and compromise of the cord.

Angiography is used less often than previously because of the advantages of computed tomography. However, it is better at showing vascular anatomy and may allow therapeutic embolisation to be performed.

14 ROLE OF THE TRAUMA NURSE

Lisa Hadfield-Law, Andrew Kent

Accident and emergency staff are responsible for receiving trauma patients at the hospital. To perform well, staff should be organised into a formal "trauma team".

To work well teams need organisation and training, a coordinated approach subscribed to by all members, and mutual trust and respect. It has been suggested that one of the best ways to develop this is to share learning programmes. Certainly team members should share mutual philosophies and adhere to the same principles of management. Recently staff in accident departments have been organising themselves into well disciplined teams in which each member carries out individual tasks simultaneously. Such roles must, however, be clearly defined because trauma nurses can assume responsibility for several areas.

- Planning
- Assessment, intervention, and evaluation
- Communication
- Documentation
- Evaluation
- Advocacy
- Debriefing

Planning

Planning is essential for all team work. Before any patient with multiple injuries arrives at the hospital a suitable environment must have been prepared. Structural aspects must be considered, together with health and safety. The orientation of new staff must be carefully planned and all relevant equipment must be checked and ready to use.

While resuscitation is in progress the nurse must stay one step ahead of the rest of the team. Valuable time will be saved if the patient's needs and eventual destination are anticipated.

Assessment, intervention, and evaluation

The nurse is usually the first member of the team to receive the patient into the hospital, and is the one person who will remain with the patient throughout his stay in the accident department and during transfer for definitive care. The trauma nurse must therefore be able to make a rapid initial assessment.

It is the trauma nurse who is in an excellent position to pick up the subtle changes in the patient's condition that indicate response to injury and to treatment.

Duties of the nursing team

In larger accident units the trauma nursing team may have as many as five members, but even with fewer there are defined areas of responsibility: leadership, airway and cervical spine, circulation, documentation, and relatives.

Types of nurse roles

- Team leadership
- Airway and cervical spine
- Circulation
- Documentation
- Relatives

Team leader

This nurse must be experienced clinically and have been specifically and appropriately trained. During the phase before the patient arrives the leader should liaise with other team members and with the medical team. The leader should be aware of colleagues' abilities and limitations, and be able to recognise signs of stress. This coordinating role should allow the nurse to maintain a "hands off" approach and maintain an overall view of the resuscitation attempt. The leader is also responsible for the health and safety of the team and should ensure that all team members are wearing protective clothing including gloves, aprons, and eye protection. It is essential that staff support systems be in place to help team members cope with the demands made on them. Constant and effective liaison with all the team members is the key to success in this role.

Airway nurse

During the patient's prehospital care the airway nurse, together with her or his medical counterpart, ensures that all equipment for management of the airway is available and working. It is helpful if the airway nurse has already been working in the resuscitation room and is familiar with the equipment and any problems with it. When the patient arrives this nurse is responsible for immobilisation of the cervical spine and with the team leader will coordinate the lift on to the trolley to take charge of the spine. After the medical assessment the airway nurse will maintain a patent airway and help the doctor concerned to initiate definitive procedures to this end, including immobilisation of the neck during intubation, or assisting in any surgical intervention.

Because of location this nurse will be responsible for talking to the patient and giving support. This aspect of her role is vital both for conscious and unconscious patients.

Circulation nurse

The role of the circulation nurse overlaps with that of the doctor. Since the publication of *The scope of professional practice*, more nurses are practising clinical skills such as intravenous cannulation which have in the past been the responsibility of the doctor.

Before the patient arrives in the accident department the nurse ensures that the intravenous fluids are warmed and the giving sets are primed so that resuscitation can be started promptly. The circulation nurse may assist doctors to insert intravenous lines or take responsibility for the insertion of one or both lines. Fluid replacement will then be given according to local policy.

The circulation nurse will also help the documentation nurse to remove the patient's clothing so that a primary survey can be made. Clothes should be removed in the safest and most painless way; cutting may not be the best way if the clothes are thick or expensive, and the patient is conscious.

The nurse should then record the baseline observations—temperature, pulse, respiration, blood pressure and cardiac monitoring—and then pass the information on to the documentation nurse. She or he should then prepare other equipment that may be needed—for example, a chest drain, or peritoneal lavage set. This should be done carefully to avoid accidental contamination. It is vital that the circulation and documentation nurses should maintain close contact as information about practical procedures and fluids and drugs given, is necessary for continuing patient care and for audit. All drugs including analgesics are arranged and given by the circulation nurse.

The circulation nurse often has the most demanding role in the team, and in some departments two nurses may share the tasks.

If it is local policy for the accident department to assist with prehospital care (see chapters 20, 21) the circulation nurse should attend the scene with the appropriate medical staff. The nurse can then go with the patient into the resuscitation room to provide continuity of care for the patient and assist in the handover of information.

If the nurse is to attend the scene of the accident she or he should be appropriately trained and have the *Prehospital trauma life support certificate* or the *Prehospital emergency care certificate*. Some local training with both the ambulance and fire service is essential. Such additional training also promotes confidence in staff members, permitting them to be effective in assessment and treatment.

Documentation nurse (scribe)

This nurse should stay away from the clinical activity and concentrate solely on recording information. If the information is not documented comprehensively and accurately the team will have difficulty in evaluating the care provided. This in turn will make decisions about definitive care difficult. Various methods can be used, ranging from a plain white board to a specially designed trauma assessment sheet. The latter allows the recording on one sheet of paper the patient's progress from the site of the accident to definitive care.

All observations made and drugs given inside and outside the hospital should be recorded in a way that is universally understood. Total fluids given should be recorded alongside fluid losses. The documentation nurse should liaise with nurses outside the resuscitation area so that blood samples can be taken to the laboratory for investigation and blood for transfusion.

All the patient's property and valuables should be taken into safe keeping by the nurse, according to the hospital protocol. This role can be taken by a less experienced member of the team who may use the opportunity to learn from more experienced nurses.

Documentation during resuscitation is often given low priority despite its importance. Patients' notes provide a record of clinical care, data for audit and research, and evidence in the event of medicolegal action. All records should provide a comprehensive chronological record of the case, responses to treatment, and the means to review the quality of care.

To gather comprehensive and accurate data this nurse should remain with the patient throughout resuscitation until definitive care starts. She or he is in an excellent position to complete all required documentation.

Relatives' nurse

By allocating one nurse to care for the relatives stress and confusion can be reduced. The nurse can, however, find the role emotionally draining, particularly if she or he has to break bad news. The nurse should meet the ambulance and accompany any relatives to a quiet area near the resuscitation room so that the patient can be transferred rapidly.

Members of the trauma team should decide beforehand whether they will be comfortable if relatives accompany patients into the resuscitation room. This issue has been successfully dealt with by staff at the Foote Hospital in Jackson, Florida, USA, who permit "selected families" to be present in the resuscitation room. This seems to give benefit to grieving families and gives them the feeling that they have been able to help the patient in some way. There is evidence that once such an approach is established both patients and staff benefit.

If the relatives have not arrived with the patient or are patients themselves in the same department, the role of the nurse is one of coordinator. She or he will keep in touch with relatives outside the hospital, and liaise with other emergency services to make sure that all relatives have been contacted. On arrival, therefore, they will be met by a nurse who is fully briefed and prepared. It is important that this nurse remains with the relatives when medical staff talk to them so that continuity of care is assured. The nurse can make sure that the relatives understand what is discussed and clarify the medical terms.

Debriefing

People working with the emergency services are particularly vulnerable to stress. Stress-related symptoms cause people to take time off work and leave the specialty for areas in which the pressure is reduced. This can be prevented if steps are taken early enough.

Stress is a state of physiological and psychological arousal as the result of threats, challenge, or change. Members of the trauma team respond normally and naturally to protect, maintain, and enhance life. Understanding physical, mental, and emotional responses can help us to use stress positively and reduce its effects by acquiring and sharing the necessary technical, human, and supervisory skills. An excellent way of alleviating stress is by debriefing or "defusing" sessions after difficult cases.

Summary

Trauma teams can be effective only if individual members have clear responsibilities. Members should be specially trained and versatile so that they can take different roles depending on the circumstances. Reductions in staff, particularly at night, can be difficult to assimilate into the team structure, and certain roles (for example, leader and airway nurses) may have to be merged if there are not enough staff.

Structured and organised teams with predetermined roles and responsibilities for both nursing and medical staff have a direct bearing on outcome for patients.

15 SCORING SYSTEMS

D W Yates

Previous chapters have emphasised the importance of an aggressive, integrated, interdisciplinary approach to trauma care by an experienced team that has immediate access to operating theatres and intensive care facilities. Many of the recommendations can be expected to incur appreciable additional costs. Will this money be well spent? Which changes are most effective in improving patient care and are there any which produce unexpected delays or complications?

To answer these questions about a system which has to respond to patients with an almost infinite constellation of injuries is a major challenge in clinical measurement and audit. Clearly, statistical analysis must replace anecdote and dogma, but the complexity of the task should not be underestimated.

The effects of injury may be defined in terms of input—an anatomical component and the physiological response—and output—mortality and morbidity. These must be coded numerically before we can comment with confidence on treatment. Elderly people and young children survive trauma less well than others, so age must be taken into account. The mechanism of injury is also important: the effect of a blunt impact from a fall or a car crash is quite different from that of a stab or gunshot wound. Most work has been concerned with the measurement of injury severity in relation to mortality, but there are two seriously impaired survivors for every person who dies of trauma and until recently the assessment of morbidity has been largely neglected.

Cost-benefit analysis of trauma care

Input
Anatomical injury
Physiological derangement

Treatment
Variations in the system of care
Variations in patient care

Output
Survival: alive or dead?
Disability: temporary or permanent?
 Neurological?
 Musculoskeletal?
 Visceral?

Input criteria

Anatomical scoring system

The *abbreviated injury scale* (AIS) was first published in 1969. It scores from 1 (minor) to 6 (fatal) over 1200 injuries, which are listed in a booklet that is now in its fourth edition. (Copies of the booklet AIS90 may be obtained from the North Western Injury Research Centre—see footnote.) The intervals between the scores are not always consistent—for example, the difference between AIS3 and AIS4 is not necessarily the same as the difference between AIS1 and AIS2—but the higher the score the worse the injury.

Examples of injuries scored by abbreviated injury scale

Injury	Score
Shoulder pain (no injury specified)	0
Wrist sprain	1 (Minor)
Closed undisplaced tibial fracture	2 (Moderate)
Head injury—unconscious on admission but for less than one hour thereafter, no neurological deficit	3 (Serious)
Major liver laceration, no loss of tissue	4 (Severe)
Incomplete transection of the thoracic aorta	5 (Critical)
Laceration of the brain stem	6 (Fatal)

Patients with multiple injuries are scored by adding together the squares of the three highest abbreviated injury scale scores in predetermined regions of the body (see box). This is the *injury severity score* (ISS). The maximum score is 75 ($5^2 + 5^2 + 5^2$). By convention a patient with an AIS6 in one body region is given an injury severity score of 75. The injury severity score is non-linear: there is pronounced variation in the frequency of different scores—9 and 16 are common, 14 and 22 unusual, and 7 and 15 unattainable. The overall injury severity score of a group of patients should be identified by the median value and the range, not the mean value. Non-parametric statistics should be used for analyses.

Injury severity score

To obtain this:
(1) Use the AIS90 dictionary to score every injury

(2) Identify the highest abbreviated injury scale score in each of the following six areas: head and neck, abdomen and pelvic contents, bony pelvis and limbs, face, chest, and body surface

(3) Add together the squares of the three highest area scores

---

Scoring systems

Case study

A man is injured in a fall at work. He complains of pain in his neck, jaw, and left wrist and has difficulty breathing. There are abrasions around the left shoulder, left side of the chest, and left knee. Examination of the cervical spine (with radiography) suggests no abnormality. There are fractures of the body of the mandible, left wrist, and left ribs (5 to 9), with a flail segment.

$$ISS = 2^2 + 2^2 + 4^2 = 24$$

Injury	Abbreviated injury scale
Fracture of body of mandible	2
Fracture of lower end of radius (not further specified*)	2
Fracture of ribs 5–9 with flail segment	4
Abrasions (all sites)	1
Neck pain†	0

* If fracture of radius was known to be displaced or open the AIS would be 3. If not specified the lower score is used.
† Symptoms are not scored if there is no demonstrable anatomical injury.

Glasgow coma scale

	Score
Eyes open:	
Spontaneously	4
To speech	3
To pain	2
Never	1
Best motor response:	
Obeys commands	6
Localises pain	5
Flexion withdrawal	4
Decerebrate flexion	3
Decerebrate extension	2
No response	1
Best verbal response:	
Orientated	5
Confused	4
Inappropriate words	3
Incomprehensible sounds	2
Silent	1

Physiological scoring systems

The *Glasgow coma scale* (GCS) is the accepted international standard for measuring neurological state. The score may be represented as a single figure (for example, GCS = 15) or as the response in each of the three sections (for example, eyes, motor response, and verbal response = 4, 6, 5). Coma is defined as a Glasgow coma scale score of < 8.

Various modifications of the scale have been suggested for use in small children. Some doctors reduce the maximum score to that which is consistent with neurological maturation. A more useful clinical device, which ensures more accurate communication and simplifies epidemiological research is to retain the maximum score of 15 but to redefine the descriptions.

Modification of Glasgow coma scale for children

	Score
Best verbal response:	
Appropriate words or social smiles, fixes on and follows objects	5
Cries but is consolable	4
Persistently irritable	3
Restless, agitated	2
Silent	1
Eye and motor responses are scored as in scale for adults	

The *revised trauma score* combines coded measurements of respiratory rate, systolic blood pressure, and Glasgow coma scale to provide a general assessment of physiological derangement. It was derived from statistical analysis of a large North American database to determine the most predictive independent outcome variables. Selection of variables was also influenced by their ease of measurement and clinical opinion. The coded value is multiplied by a weighting factor derived from regression analysis of the database. This correction reflects the relative value of the measurement in determining survival.

The injury severity score is often underestimated when the patient first arrives at hospital, and the revised trauma score changes as resuscitation progresses. For the purposes of the analyses described below the injury severity score should be calculated only from operative findings, appropriate investigations, or necropsy reports. The revised trauma score is, by convention, taken as the score recorded when the patient first arrives in the accident and emergency department.

Revised trauma score

	Coded value	× weighting factor	= score
Respiratory rate (breaths/min):			
10–29	4		
>29	3		
6–9	2	0.2908	_____
1–5	1		
0	0		
Systolic blood pressure (mm Hg):			
>89	4		
76–89	3		
50–75	2	0.7326	_____
1–49	1		
0	0		
Glasgow coma scale:			
13–15	4		
9–12	3		
6–8	2	0.9368	_____
4–5	1		
3	0		
	Total = revised trauma score:		_____

TRISS methodology

Probability of survival of individual patient

$$P) = \frac{1}{1 + e^{-b}}$$

Where e = natural logarithm and
$b = b_0 + b_1 (RTS) + b_2(ISS) + b_3(A)$
b_0–b_3 are weighted coefficients based on major trauma outcome study (UK) data. These differ for blunt and penetrating injuries
RTS = revised trauma score
ISS = injury severity score
A = age (score 0 if $\leq$ 54, score 1 if $\geq$ 55)

Population outcome comparison
Ws statistic measures difference between actual and predicted number of deaths or survivors standardised to account for variations in injury severity (number per 100 patients)
Zs statistic measures statistical significance of Ws (NS – 1.96 to + 1.96)

Hospital review

Example
St Elsewhere District General Hospital treated 739 patients in one year who fulfilled the entry requirements for the major trauma outcome study. 677 patients survived. A survival probability is calculated for each patient using TRISS. The expected number of survivors in each Ps band is calculated by summing the individual survival probabilities. These were distributed in 6 Ps bands as follows:

Ps	Total patients	Survivors	Predicted to survive
1.00–0.96	636	626	625.3
0.95–0.91	31	25	29.0
0.90–0.76	19	11	16.0
0.75–0.51	31	13	19.9
0.50–0.26	9	2	3.6
0.25–0.00	13	0	0.8
	739	677	694.6

The W score for each Ps band is then calculated.
For example, for the Ps 1.00—0.96 band:

$$W = \frac{626 - 625.3}{636/100} = 0.11$$

This W is then multiplied by the fraction of patients in this band on the national dataset:

$$0.11 \times 0.885 = 0.10$$

Similar calculations are performed for each Ps interval and all six products added to give a standardised W or "Ws"
In this example Ws = 1.93.
This indicates that at this hospital it is estimated that for every 100 trauma patients seen about two more deaths are occurring than would be expected in a typical UK hospital which returns data to the major trauma outcome study.

The degree of physiological derangement and the extent of the anatomical injury are measures of the threat to life. Mortality will also be affected by the age of the patient and by the method of wounding. A blunt assault produces different injury characteristics and physiological abnormalities than does a penetrating object.

The "TRISS methodology" combines the four elements—revised trauma score, injury severity score, age of the patient, and whether the injury is blunt or penetrating—to provide a measure of the probability of survival (Ps). (The acronym is tortuously developed from **TR**auma score and **I**njury **S**everity **S**core.) It is important to appreciate that Ps is merely a mathematical calculation; it is not an absolute measure of mortality but only of the probability of death. If a patient with a Ps of 80% dies the outcome is unexpected in that four out of five patients with such a Ps could be expected to survive. But the fifth would be expected to die—and this could be the patient under study. The use of charts to identify patients whose Ps lies on the "wrong side" of a line that represents 50% mortality is widespread but may lead to inappropriate conclusions being drawn about the care of individual patients if this point is not recognised. Such charts are helpful in identifying patients for discussion at audit meetings but should not be used as the sole measure of performance.

Case study

A 65 year old pedestrian is knocked down, sustaining head, abdominal, and leg injuries. On arrival in the accident and emergency department he has a Glasgow coma score of 9, respiratory rate of 35 beats/min, and systolic blood pressure of 80 mm Hg. Computed tomography shows a small subdural haematoma with swelling of the left parietal lobe.. There is a major laceration of the liver but no other intra-abdominal injury. Radiographs of the lower limbs show displaced fractures through both upper tibias.

Revised trauma score:
Glasgow coma score = 9; coded value 3 × weighting 0.9368 = 2.8104
Respiratory rate = 35; coded value 3 × weighting 0.2908 = 0.8724
Blood pressure = 80; coded value 3 × weighting 0.7326 = 2.1978
RTS = 5.8806

Injury severity score

	Abbreviated injury score
Subdural haematoma (small)	4
[Parietal lobe swelling]	[3]
Liver laceration (major)	4
Upper tibial fracture (displaced)	3

$$ISS = 4^2 + 4^2 + 3^2 = 41$$

Probability of survival
Coefficients from major trauma outcome study database for blunt injury:
$b_0 = 0.945$
$b_1 = 0.642$
$b_2 = -0.122$
$b_3 = -1.886$

$$b = 0.945 + (0.642)(5.8806) + (-0.122)(41) + (-1.886)(1)$$

$$P_s = \frac{1}{1 + e^{-(-2.1677)}} = 0.103$$

Probability of survival = 10·3%

Major trauma outcome study

The major trauma outcome study

— Measures overall severity of injury
— Records management and outcome
— Provides a database for audit in individual patients
— Allows comparison of performance over time and between hospitals

First developed in North America, the method employed in the major trauma outcome study is now also used in the United Kingdom and Europe to audit the effectiveness of systems of trauma care and the management of individual patients. The TRISS methodology is applied in all patients with trauma who are admitted to hospital for more than three days, managed in an intensive care area, referred for specialist care, or die in hospital. Additional information is sought about pre hospital care, the seniority of doctors attending the patient on arrival at hospital, the initial management, and the timing of consultations and operations.

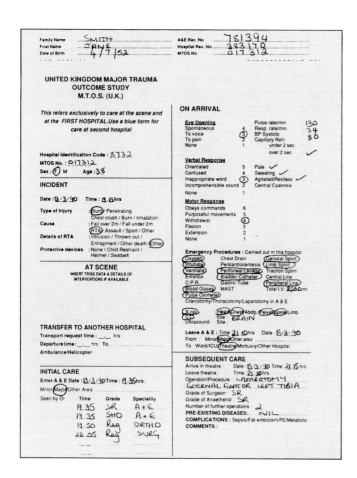

Output variables

Validation of the recently published Injury Impairment Scale is required before it can be used in clinical audit

Measurement of the change in mortality that may occur in patients with a given combination of anatomical injury and physiological derangement is only one method of assessing the effects of modifications in the system of care. The quality of life of the survivors may vary considerably. The Glasgow outcome score is a recognised method for measuring the severity of permanent neurological impairment. Overall impairment, particularly in relation to musculoskeletal problems is more difficult to measure. An Injury Impairment Scale has recently been published by the authors of the Abbreviated Injury Scale but has yet to be validated against a large database. (Copies may be obtained from the North Western Injury Research Centre, see footnote.)

Future developments

Objectives of scoring systems

Short term objectives
- Better prehospital data
- Consistent hospital scoring
- Improved necropsy reports

Long term objectives

More sensitive scales to include:

- Biomechanical measurements
- More sensitive physiological assessment
- Biochemical analyses
- Assessment of temporary and permanent morbidity

Definitions of impairment, disability, and handicap

Impairment has an anatomical or physiological basis and is usually a consequence of musculoskeletal or cerebral injury (for example, an amputated finger, anosmia). It is easy to measure but variably related to the patient's activity

Disability is a functional consequence of an impairment so that the patient cannot perform activities of daily life. Its measurement is relevant to the patient's needs but it is influenced by the environment

Handicap refers to disability within the patient's social and professional environment. It reflects a change in lifestyle, but it is difficult to relate it to specific injury and is very difficult to measure

There are wide variations in the provision of emergency medical services throughout the world, and the optimal system for the United Kingdom is still under debate. The major trauma outcome study provides an invaluable method for comparing the patterns of care in different parts of the country. This can be achieved only if data are carefully collected in a consistent format to allow collation and comparison of results. Deaths caused by trauma are too varied, too complicated, and too important to be discussed in isolation in individual hospitals, however sophisticated their software. The wide perspective of the major trauma outcome study is increasingly recognised as the only valid approach to trauma audit and is being taken up by regional and national bodies for this purpose. Identification of deficiencies is valuable, however, only if a mechanism exists to correct them. Local audit meetings and national comparisons must be used to stimulate appropriate changes in the systems of trauma care.

The development of the TRISS methodology has been a major advance in the measurement of injury severity. The detailed structure of the scales, particularly the neurological component of the abbreviated injury scale, the calculation of the injury severity score and the composition of the revised trauma score, continue to attract interest.

Further developments can be expected to lead to more accurate scoring systems, but for the present the TRISS methodology has a worldwide reputation for consistency and reasonable prediction of outcome. Immediate improvements in its usefulness could be made if, as is happening in some areas, ambulance crews measured the revised trauma score at the scene of the accident. This would allow a more scientific appraisal of the value of prehospital care. The accuracy of anatomical information could also be improved—particularly in necropsy reports: these are often inadequate for coding purposes and spinal cord injuries are rarely described in detail.

The latest edition of the *Abbreviated Injury Scale Booklet* (AIS90), the Injury Impairment Scale, and information about the major trauma outcome study (UK) are available from the North Western Injury Research Centre, University of Manchester, Hope Hospital, Salford M6 8HD.

16 HANDLING DISTRESSED RELATIVES AND BREAKING BAD NEWS

C A J McLauchlan

Coping with major trauma is stressful for both staff and relatives. Handling distressed relatives is an underemphasised part of the work, and medical staff may have had no training and little experience of it. It is a time that the relative will always remember and, if handled badly, will leave lasting scars. Alternatively, skilled early handling of the bereaved will enable them to make a smoother journey through grief and improve the long term outlook.

Giving bad news is never easy, but it can be especially difficult in cases of major trauma when there is physical damage to the loved one. The nature of the patient's problem and the bad news can be varied. The management of the relatives may begin before they arrive at hospital and carry on until well after death or discharge of the patient. The principles of management apply to the accident and emergency department as well as the intensive treatment unit or admitting ward. Providing genuine care and support for relatives is the key to their management.

Initial contact

When a victim of major trauma arrives in the emergency room the priority is immediate resuscitation. Once identified, the closest relatives or friends should be notified.

Communication with the emergency services can provide important information that is useful when handling the relatives. The ambulance crew and police, as well as giving details about the incident, may have already seen the relatives or know their whereabouts. It is usually better for a sympathetic police officer to make the initial contact in person rather than for a telephone call to be made from the hospital, but local knowledge may be important. The police may also be able to help with transport.

If the telephone is used information should be given by an experienced nurse or doctor and a lone relative advised strongly against driving to hospital alone. Mentioning that the victim is unconscious often helps to impart a certain severity to the lay person, although the full severity or death is usually best explained in person at the hospital. If relatives are not told of the victim's death, however, they may blame themselves for not arriving at the hospital in time to be with their loved one at death. It is important to dispel any self recrimination by giving the relatives the exact information, including the time of death, when they attend. If the relatives have to travel great distances or from overseas the full details, including death, may have to be explained over the telephone. Find out if the relative is alone and, if so, suggest that he or she seeks support locally. Offer to telephone for support.

Arrival of relatives at the hospital

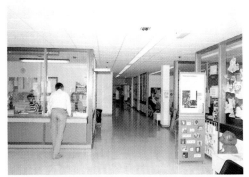

Distressed relatives should be given privacy and not kept waiting in reception areas, which may be impersonal and busy.

Anxious relatives should be met by a named link nurse and not be kept waiting around at reception for the department's or ward's communications to be established. Therefore, it is important that the nursing sister coordinates the information so that the staff, in particular those at reception, know that potentially distressed relatives are expected. They should be welcomed and not made to feel in the way. Staff should remember that it is not only the victim's relatives who may be distressed: in some instances close friends or partners of either sex may be severely distressed and should be handled in the same way as the relatives.

There should be a private room or office where relatives and friends can wait and be seen. Ideally this room should be solely for relatives and friends, have a homely decor, yet be nearby and not isolated. An outside view is desirable, or at least a controlled view of a corridor. It is a myth that such details are not remembered by distressed relatives.

Breaking the news

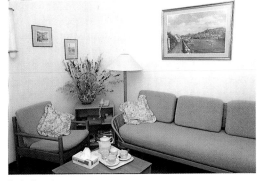

Relatives' room

Remember to ask relatives for the medical history of the patient. This history may be vital if the patient is receiving certain drugs such as steroids or anticoagulants, and an idea of the quality of life may be useful in elderly victims or those with disease. Providing a history can also make relatives feel that they are doing something.

During attempted resuscitation relatives should at least be given early warning if the condition is critical. Regular updates by the same person (usually the link nurse) are also appreciated and may help to break the bad news in stages. It also allows relationships to form, which will help in providing the support that may be needed later.

The link nurse should introduce a doctor, preferably a senior one to the relatives as soon as possible to provide further information. There are no firm rules as to who should break the news, but ideally it should be someone senior with the time, warmth, and communication skills. Relatives will expect to see a doctor for medical information and an idea of the prognosis: "Will he be all right, doctor?"

Advice for the doctor (or other breaker of news)

Breaking bad news has to be tailored to the situation and the particular relatives, but the following principles generally apply:

- On leaving the resuscitation area or theatre you may be stressed, so take a moment to compose yourself and think about what you are going to say while you take a few deep breaths. Also remove evidence of blood stains, etc, so that you are physically and mentally prepared

- Take an experienced nurse with you. The link nurse can be a great support and can carry on where you leave off

- Confirm that you have the correct relatives. Briefly ascertain what information they already have

- Enter the relatives' room, introduce yourself, and sit down near the patient's closest relative at eye level. Do not stand holding the door handle like a bus conductor ready to jump out. Giving the impression that you have time to talk and listen is important

- In general look at who you are talking to, be honest and direct, and keep it simple. Be prepared to emphasise the main points. Avoid too much technical information at this stage (although with patients with multiple injuries there may be much going on). If death is probable say so; do not beat about the bush

- After breaking bad news allow time and silence while the facts sink in

- If the seriousness of the situation does not seem to have been accepted, re-emphasise the facts and consider showing them the patient or deceased person immediately

- Be prepared for a variety of emotional responses or reactions. Some people may stick at one reaction whereas others go through several reactions. These reactions are not your fault—rather they imply that you have got the message over

Handling distressed relatives and breaking bad news

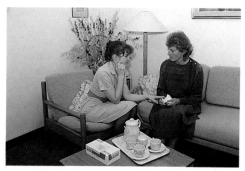
A sensitive nurse is a great asset after the news has been broken.

- Allow and encourage reactions such as crying. Provide tissues and facilities for relatives to make themselves presentable to the world again
- Although it is upsetting, close relatives appreciate the truth and your honest empathy
- At this stage there is no substitute for genuine care and support. A sensitive nurse is a great asset
- Tea usually appears, and this is another sign that the relatives' distress is appreciated
- During the interview it is a helpful and natural comfort for staff to touch or hold the hand of the relative. Various social and cultural factors may influence the appropriateness of touching, but generally if it feels right then it is probably right
- Likewise, during the interview it may be natural for the staff to have sad feelings, and these need not be completely hidden. Some sign of emotion may help distressed or bereaved people to realise that the staff do have some understanding and it is not just another case
- Avoid platitudes—for example, after a death comments such as "you've still got your other son, etc," which are not helpful as it is the dead person whom the relatives want back. Also avoid false sympathy as in "I know what it's like," but rather empathise, as in: "It must be hard for you . . ." or "It must feel very unreal and a shock for you . . .," etc, reflecting back their emotions.

Encourage and be prepared for questions to be asked during the interview. These may disclose any misunderstandings and present a chance to re-emphasise the message. The question of pain and suffering is common and should be discussed routinely, with reassurance as appropriate. The prognosis may be unknown initially, and you should say so. If death or serious disability is possible, however, then it is only fair to be honest and warn the relatives. It will be a worse shock later if they have been protected from this knowledge. Do not be afraid to answer that you do not know the answers to medical or philosophical questions such as "Why me?" Other difficult questions may arise from feelings of guilt or when a relative was involved in but not injured in the same accident. Special problems may arise if the relative feels responsible directly—for example, as the driver in an accident. Other complications may include a recent squabble before the accident with subsequent self recrimination. The "If only . . ." rumination can be a type of guilt response that is fruitless and should be understood but discouraged at the outset. Just listening may be all that is needed.

If death has already occurred the same principles as discussed above apply. It is important to use the word "death" or "dead" early and avoid euphemisms such as "passed on" or "lost", which can be misinterpreted. The news is usually hard to accept and so it must be as clear as possible, abrupt as it may seem. People usually need an explanation as to the cause of death of a loved one. It may be helpful to explain the inevitability in the light of known injuries and that "everything possible was done". Worries about their own first aid at the scene of the accident may need talking through.

Children should not be excluded from the proceedings in the mistaken belief that they need protection. They will be afraid and may have fantasies and feelings of guilt needing more information and listening to rather than less. Parents and carers may need support and explanation about a child's or teenager's reaction.

Staff actions during the interview with the bereaved

Allow
- Time
- The bereaved to react
- Silence
- Touching
- Questions

Avoid
- Rushing
- "Protecting" from the truth
- Platitudes
- False sympathy
- Euphemisms
- Talking instead of listening

Whenever possible relatives should be given a clear explanation of the cause of death

---

Management of relatives

Reality is preferable to fantasy so allow relatives to see even critically ill patients, albeit briefly

Seeing the patient

Depending on the urgency of further treatment it should be possible as well as beneficial for close relatives to see the patient briefly before he or she is rushed off to theatre, the intensive treatment unit, or even another hospital. Although distressing, reality is usually preferable to fantasy. Also, sometimes this may be the last time that they will see their loved one alive and this contact may be beneficial to the conscious patient. Relatives may ask to enter or remain in the resuscitation area during emergency treatment, especially of infants and children. This is not yet generally accepted except in some paediatric units, but it seems that it can be beneficial provided that they are supported by an advocate such as the link nurse, and the relatives want to be there (a relative may better appreciate both the seriousness of the situation and the vigour of resuscitation efforts).[1] Hospital staff may, however, be apprehensive about the presence of relatives and the concept should be introduced gently although the prime consideration must be the relatives' wishes. Certainly staff should respond promptly to any request to see a dying patient or a dead person.

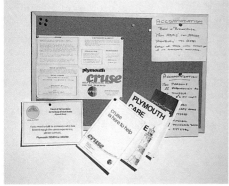

Useful information in the relatives' room.

Seeing the body after death

The opportunity to see the dead person should always be offered and gently encouraged if there is any doubt. Well meaning friends may try and discourage this act, which is an important part of accepting reality, and relatives may also like to see the place of death.

The imagination is usually far worse than reality, and cruel fantasies about the victim being disfigured or squashed flat can be dispelled. The actions and words of staff when relatives are with the body should give "permission" for relatives to touch, hold, kiss, or say goodbye to their loved one. Staff will often carefully prepare a body before viewing in the clinical area or chapel. Ideally there should be a private cubicle near the resuscitation area, made as non-clinical as possible, to allow relatives time with the deceased person. There should also be a non-religious "chapel of rest" for later opportunities for visiting. Religious insignia can be added as appropriate. The relative may also like to be left alone with the body and must be given permission to stay as long as they wish or is practically possible.

Checklist of actions in the event of death

- Notify the general practitioner, other relatives and friends, and the coroner's officer
- Ensure that the minister or chaplain has been called if the relatives wish and any religious or ethnic issues considered
- Give an information or help leaflet to the relatives
- Notify the social worker if he or she is available
- Give useful telephone numbers and contact addresses (and your name) to the relatives

Other actions

Although they are stunned by events, it is often the small touches of care that relatives appreciate and remember, such as being given a lock of hair from their dead child (or adult relative) by a thoughtful nurse.

Always ask if there is anyone else whom the relatives would like to be contacted—for example, a close friend or a minister. The relatives or appropriate minister should be consulted about any religious or ethnic issues and the correct procedures. Staff should be aware of the main minority groups in their area. The hospital chaplains can be a source of great support to both relatives and busy staff.

The patient's wishes regarding organ donation can be raised sensitively, particularly if a donor card is found. Corneas and heart valves can be donated up to 24 hours after death.

If a mechanism of counselling and follow up exists locally consider borrowing their expertise in appropriate cases of trauma.

Sedation may be requested for relatives, usually by a third party but is generally inappropriate as it dulls reality and may delay acceptance. Grieving cannot be avoided so easily.

Information and follow up

Long term management and bereavement counselling is not within the scope of this article, but arrangements for follow up may need initiating on day one. If the nurse or doctor concerned in the emergency department feels able they can offer to be available for any questions later. Some departments have a social worker who can provide some practical help as well as coordinate follow up. If death occurs it is helpful to have a routine checklist, which includes notifying the general practitioner. An open invitation can be posted to the relatives to offer an interview with a consultant so that questions on the events or necropsy findings can be answered. Many take up this offer, sometimes months later, to fill in gaps in their information which helps them to make some sense of it.

An up to date leaflet explaining official procedures slipped into a relative's pocket is useful for later perusal (for example, leaflet D49, *What to do after Death*, which is published by the Department of Health). Participation by the Coroner's officer, who may be a policeman, should be explained. Warning relatives of the possibility of

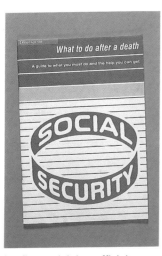

Leaflet explaining official procedures after death.

them developing symptoms of post-traumatic stress disorder is appropriate in certain cases. Such symptoms include depression, anxiety, and flash backs, with a wide range of severity. Also, it may be necessary in follow up to warn them of possible avoiding or unhelpful actions by neighbours. A local leaflet explaining possible reactions as well as local information on the Coroner, registration of death and funeral should also be provided. Details of any support organisations such as CRUSE, RoadPeace or any local groups should be included.

Staff's reaction

Lastly, do not forget the carers. There are many different reactions, the commonest of which are sadness, anger, and guilt.[2] Staff including the ambulance crew may identify with particular people or situations. For example, a child being killed will be particularly upsetting, especially for staff with children of the same age. Part of the debriefing on major trauma must include an opportunity for members of staff to express their feelings. In emergency areas this is usually done informally at coffee or handover but formal mechanisms of staff support should also exist. Hiding behind a defence of excessive concern with composure or tasks should be avoided. Late feedback on the patient's progress or necropsy is also helpful and provides a further opportunity for discussion.

Difficulties for hospital staff in breaking bad news

- Lack of training and experience
- Fear of being blamed
- Not knowing how to cope with relatives' reactions
- Fear of expressing emotion
- Fear of not knowing the answers
- Fear of their own death or disability

Conclusion

National contact addresses

- **CRUSE** (for care of the bereaved) Cruse House, 126 Sheen Road, Richmond, Surrey TW9 1UR. Tel 0171 940 4818
- **Compassionate Friends** (for bereaved parents) 6 Denmark Street, Bristol BS1 5DQ. Tel 0117 9292778
- **Foundation for the Study of Infant Deaths** 15 Belgrave Square, London SW1X 8PS. Tel 0171 235 1721
- **Samaritans** (for the despairing) 17 Uxbridge Road, Slough SL1 1SN. Tel 01753 32713
- **RoadPeace** (Information and support after deaths on the road) PO Box 2579, London NW10 3PW. Tel 0181 964 1021

Because of its suddenness and severity major trauma is especially difficult to cope with for relatives and staff. However bad the news is relatives need direct, honest information along with genuine care and support. Many doctors find this important part of their work difficult. Reasons have been suggested for this.[3] Awareness may help the situation and lead to a greater emphasis in training.

In short, the principles of dealing with the distressed relative can be remembered as follows:

- **Empathise.** Sit, listen, and reflect back relatives' reactions rather than make assumptions or categorise them
- **Enable** relatives to accept reality and the pain with honesty and easy access to their loved one
- **Encourage,** as in "you will be able to cope" (with help if needed)
- **Encounter** your own feelings and express them later, perhaps as part of a debriefing.

1 Doyle C, Post H, Burney R, Maino J, Keefe M, Rhea K. Family participation during resuscitation: an option. *Ann Emerg Med* 1987; **16**: 673–5.
2 Wright B. Sudden death: aspects which incapacitate the carer. *Nursing* 1988; **3**: 12–5.
3 Buckman R. Breaking bad news: Why is it still so difficult? *BMJ* 1984; **288**: 1597–9.

Further reading

Kübler-Ross E. *On death and dying.* New York: MacMillan, 1969.
Wright B. *Sudden death.* Edinburgh: Churchill Livingstone, 1990.

I thank Sister Susan Judge, Reverend Bob Irving, Dr Sheila Cassidy, and the staff of the accident and emergency department, Derriford Hospital, Plymouth, for ideas and advice; Jackie Eccleson for typing the manuscript; and the photographic department. I also thank the unfortunate relatives, whose reactions, comments, and questions have formed the basis of this chapter.

17 TRAUMA IN PREGNANCY

Pamela Nash, Peter Driscoll

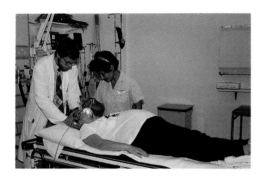

When a pregnant woman presents with trauma, two lives are at risk. Survival of the fetus depends on maternal survival. Treatment priorities remain the same as in patients who are not pregnant, although resuscitation and stabilisation should be modified to account for the anatomical and physiological changes of pregnancy. Early participation of an obstetrician and a surgeon is advocated.

If the patient is conscious she will be anxious about herself and her baby. It is important to establish rapport with her quickly. Allocation of an experienced nurse to this task will facilitate communication and allow other members of the trauma team to complete the primary and secondary surveys.

Anatomical changes

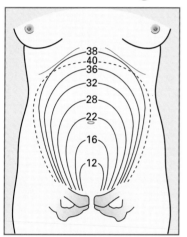

Size of uterus at various stages of pregnancy.

In the first trimester of pregnancy the fetus is protected within the thick walled uterus by the mother's pelvis. As the uterus enlarges to become an intra-abdominal organ, it becomes progressively more vulnerable to injury. The fetus is cushioned by a large volume of amniotic fluid in the second trimester but by full term there is little protection for the fetus from the relatively small volume of amniotic fluid and the thin-walled uterus. Unlike the uterine wall, the placenta is devoid of elastic tissue, so shearing forces to the abdomen—for example, those caused by blunt trauma—may cause placental abruption.

Physiological changes

Physiological changes in pregnancy

Respiratory
- Tidal volume is increased by 40%
- Respiratory rate is unchanged
- Respiratory alkalosis

Cardiovascular
- Pulse rate is increased to 85–90 beats/ minute
- Blood pressure falls by 5–15 mm Hg in second trimester
- Plasma volume is increased
- The aortocaval compression syndrome

Other changes
- Gastric emptying is delayed
- Risk of eclampsia

Airway

The airway may be compromised because of the increased risk of regurgitation and aspiration during pregnancy.

Breathing

The "physiological hyperventilation" of pregnancy results in respiratory alkalosis with P_aCO_2 at full term falling to 30 mm Hg. A $PaCO_2$ of 40 mm Hg at this stage of pregnancy indicates maternal and fetal acidosis.

Circulation

Interpretation of maternal pulse and blood pressure readings can be difficult. The fetus may be shocked before the mother develops tachycardia, tachypnoea, or hypotension, as blood is shunted away from the uteroplacental circulation to maintain maternal vital signs. In the supine position the enlarged uterus compresses the great vessels, impairing venous return and causing a fall in cardiac output of up to 40%. This may be sufficient to produce a fall in maternal blood pressure (the aortocaval compression syndrome).

During pregnancy, blood volume increases by up to 50% and cardiac output by 1.0–1.5 litres. **Compared with other patients, pregnant women have to lose more blood before signs of hypovolaemia develop.**

Primary survey

Primary survey
• **A**irway and cervical spine control
• **B**reathing
• **C**irculation (position patient to avoid supine hypotension) and control of haemorrhage
• **D**ysfunction of the central nervous system
• **E**xposure

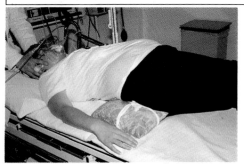

Patient with hip raised on a sandbag.

During the primary survey, life-threatening injuries to the mother are detected and treated.

Control the airway, stabilise the neck, assess ventilation, and give high flow oxygen through a mask-bag-reservoir system.

The patient should be positioned to prevent aortocaval compression. If cervical spine injury is suspected, immobilise the neck with a hard collar, sandbags, and tape, then raise the right hip on a sandbag and manually displace the uterus to the left. Once spinal injury is excluded, nurse the patient in the left lateral position.

Establish venous access with two large bore cannulas (14 gauge) in the antecubital fossas. Take blood for grouping and crossmatching and measurement of full blood count, and urea and electrolyte concentrations. Start vigorous fluid replacement with crystalloid or colloid. Haemaccel has a product licence for use in pregnant patients and can be used before crossmatched blood is available. Occasionally O negative blood is required for immediate, life saving transfusion.

If a pneumatic antishock suit is used, only the leg compartments should be inflated.

Make a rapid neurological assessment and remove all clothing.

Secondary survey

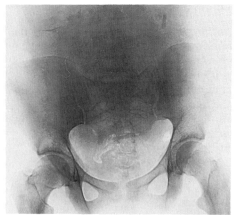

Radiograph taken after a fall excludes pelvic fracture.

Assessment of the fetus
• Note date of last menstrual period
• Measure fundal height
• Examine for uterine contractions or tenderness
• Examine for fetal movement
• Monitor fetal heart rate
• Perform vaginal examination for amniotic fluid or blood

Signs of fetal distress
• Bradycardia (<110 beats/minute)
• Signs on cardiotocography: Inadequate accelerations in fetal heart rate in response to uterine contraction Late decelerations in fetal heart rate in response to uterine contraction

Assessment of the mother

During the secondary survey the mother is examined from head to toe. Urgent radiography should not be withheld as the priority is to detect life threatening maternal injuries. The presence of a pelvic fracture should alert the clinician to the possibility of damage to the dilated pelvic veins and subsequent massive retroperitoneal haemorrhage. The radiation dose to the uterus can be reduced by keeping repeat abdominal or pelvic radiography to a minimum and using lead abdominal shields when taking peripheral *x* ray films.

Injuries should be treated in the same way as in those patients who are not pregnant. Peritoneal lavage can be done if indicated through a supraumbilical minilaparotomy after placement of a urinary catheter and nasogastric tube. Abdominal surgery should not be delayed because of pregnancy.

Assessment of the fetus

Assessment of the fetus is part of the secondary survey of the mother and should be made by an obstetrician.

Clinical examination assesses fundal height, uterine tenderness or contractions, and fetal position. Vaginal examination detects vaginal or amniotic fluid loss, cervical dilatation, and effacement.

Monitoring of fetal heart rate and pelvic ultrasonography are the most useful investigations to assess fetal wellbeing. Doppler ultrasonography can be used to auscultate the fetal heart rate from 12–14 weeks' gestation. Fetal bradycardia (less than 110 beats/minute) and loss of beat-to-beat variation are signs of fetal distress. Beyond 20 weeks' gestation the fetus may be monitored by cardiotocography, which compares fetal heart rate with uterine contractions. Signs of fetal distress include inadequate acceleration in fetal heart rate in response to uterine contractions and late decelerations in response to contractions.

Fetal gestation and viability can be confirmed by pelvic ultrasonography, the fetal heart beat being visible from seven weeks' gestation. Ultrasonography is also useful in later pregnancy to assess placental position, volume of liquor, intra-amniotic haemorrhage, and placental abruption. The Kleihauer test for fetomaternal haemorrhage has limited value in trauma because it lacks specificity. It should, however, be done for Rh negative mothers, as those with fetomaternal haemorrhage require prophylactic anti-D to protect against Rh sensitisation.

Blunt trauma

Obstetric complications of blunt trauma (%)

• Uterine Contractions	67
• Abruption	11
• Abortion/death	7
• Fetal decelerations	7
• Premature labour	4
• Vaginal bleeding	4

Signs of placental abruption

• Vaginal bleeding
• Uterine irritability
• Abdominal tenderness
• Increasing fundal height
• Maternal hypovolaemic shock
• Fetal distress

Road traffic accidents are the commonest cause of blunt trauma during pregnancy. Other causes are assaults and falls. Obstetric complications of blunt trauma include uterine contractions, placental abruption, abortion, or fetal death.

Placental abruption is a common cause of fetal death after blunt trauma, second only to maternal hypovolaemic shock. Clinical signs are usually obvious but fetal distress may be the only indicator. Cardiotocographic monitoring is advocated during the first six hours of admission to detect signs of fetal distress. Major placental separation with or without amniotic fluid embolism can lead to disseminated intravascular coagulation.

In the late stages of pregnancy, the uterus is susceptible to traumatic rupture. This has a wide range of presentations from massive haemorrhage and shock to minimal symptoms and signs. The finding of a separately palpable uterus and fetus is pathgnomonic.

Penetrating trauma

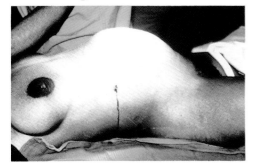

Penetrating abdominal trauma.

As pregnancy progresses the uterus becomes increasingly vulnerable to penetrating trauma, with the uterus acting as a shield for the other abdominal organs. After gunshot or stab wounds to the abdomen, fetal injury and death are common but maternal survival is good because the uterus is not a vital organ.

Burns

Immediate delivery is indicated when maternal burns exceed 50% of body surface area in the second or third trimester

The maternal mortality is high in pregnant patients in the second or third trimester who have burns of 50% or more of their body surface area. These patients should be delivered immediately as maternal death is otherwise certain and fetal prognosis is not improved by waiting.

Indications for admission

Indications for surgical or obstetric intervention

• Need for treatment of maternal injuries
• Penetrating abdominal trauma
• Uterine rupture
• Placental abruption
• Fetal distress at >26 weeks' gestation
• Burns affecting >50% of body surface area in second or third trimester
• Need for caesarean section after maternal death

Admission to a hospital with both obstetric and surgical facilities is indicated when there is vaginal bleeding or amniotic fluid loss, uterine irritability, abdominal tenderness, pain or cramps, evidence of hypovolaemia, or abnormality of fetal heart sounds.

Conclusion

The priorities in the management of pregnant women with trauma are the same as for patients who are not pregnant. The aims are to resuscitate and stabilise the mother, and then assess the fetus with the help of an obstetrician.

18 PAEDIATRIC TRAUMA

A R Lloyd-Thomas, I Anderson

Trauma is the most common cause of death in childhood, with the aetiology of the injury varying with age. Road traffic accidents and falls account for 80% of injuries.

Effective management in the first 20 minutes after an accident can do much to reduce morbidity and mortality in children with trauma. In those who reach emergency facilities alive the commonest causes of preventable death are errors in the management of ventilation and circulation and failure to detect hidden injuries. Therefore early participation of senior staff who are familiar with the surgical, anaesthetic, and medical management of children is essential.

Because children are small multisystem injury is common. Thoracic and abdominal injuries are most commonly due to major blunt trauma, and, unlike in adults, it is unusual to see penetrating injuries. Furthermore, appreciable damage to internal organs can occur without overlying bony fractures. Associated head trauma is more common.

Causes of childhood trauma

Age 0–1 years—Choking/suffocation, burns, drowning, falls

Age 1–4 years—Road traffic accidents (as occupants of vehicle), burns, drowning, falls

Age 5–14 years—Road traffic accidents (as occupant or pedestrian), bicycle injuries, burns, drowning

---

PRIMARY SURVEY

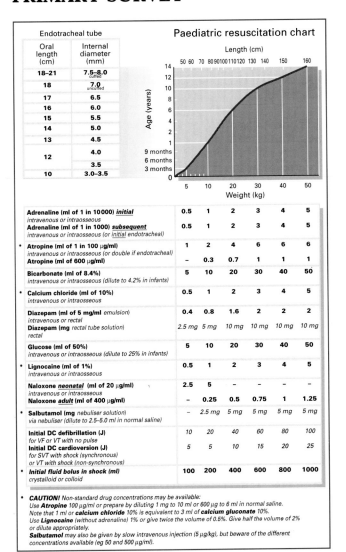

The assessment of children with multiple injuries should follow the same protocol outlined for adults. The tasks delineated in this chapter should be performed simultaneously by team members. The basic principle of resuscitation is to begin treatment of life threatening injuries immediately and not after complete evaluation of the child.

It is vital to know the weight of the child to calculate fluid volumes and drug doses. It is often impossible to weigh an injured child, but measuring head to toe length is easy, and reference to the nomogram on the paediatric resuscitation chart enables a reasonable estimate of age and weight.

Though efficient and aggressive management is essential, the conscious but injured child will be very frightened, and a team member should be allocated to give comfort and explain what is happening.

Airway management with protection of cervical spine

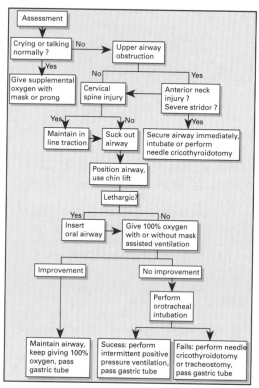

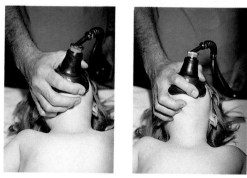

Children have specific anatomical differences compared with adults that can make maintenance of a clear airway and tracheal intubation difficult. They include:

- Large head relative to body size
- Small oral cavity with a relatively large tongue
- Large angle of the jaw (infant 140°, adult 120°)
- Epiglottis is more "U" shaped than in adults
- Larynx is cephalad (glottis at C3 in infant, C5–6 in adults) with an anterior and inferior inclination
- Cricoid ring is the narrowest part of the airway
- Trachea is short (newborn 4–5 cm, at 18 months 7–8 cm)
- Infants of 6 months or less are obligate nose breathers.

After assessment of the airway supplemental oxygen should be given to all children with trauma until further assessment shows that it is not required. Infants have a high oxygen consumption, a reduced functional residual capacity, and a high closing capacity, which leads to an increased right to left (physiological) shunt. This may be exacerbated, for example, by thoracic injury or diaphragmatic splinting due to raised intra-abdominal pressure. Nasal prongs are often better tolerated than masks by infants, but in the emergency setting they should be avoided in infants of less than six months, who are obligate nose breathers and in whom the prong may cause nasal obstruction.

If there is evidence of injury above the clavicles assume that the cervical spine has been damaged. A collar of appropriate size should be applied or, in infants, sandbags placed on either side of the head with tape across the forehead and on to a trolley to restrict head movement.

Maintaining a clear airway. (Left) Supporting fingers placed in the submental triangle causing posterior displacement of the tongue and airway obstruction. (Right) Correct placement of the hand and jaw lift.

Clearing the airway

Secretions, vomit, blood, and foreign bodies in the airway should be removed. A free airway is best maintained in children by placing the head in slight extension and pulling the mandible forward, taking care not to place the supporting fingers in the submental triangle (any pressure in this area in children results in posterior displacement of the tongue and further airway obstruction). If the patient has a gag reflex he or she should be able to maintain an airway, and insertion of an artificial airway should not be attempted as it may precipitate choking, laryngospasm, or vomiting.

Appropriate sizes and indications for use of paediatric equipment according to the age (approximate weight) of the child

Equipment	0–6 months (1–6 kg)	6–12 months (4–9 kg)	1–3 years (10–15 kg)	4–7 years (16–20 kg)	8–11 years (22–33 kg)
Airway/breathing:					
Oxygen facepiece	0	0/1	1	1/2	2/3 (Adult)
Oral airways	000/00	0/1	0/1	1/2	2
Resuscitator	Baby	Baby	Baby/adult	Adult	Adult
Breathing system	"T" piece	"T" piece	"T" piece	"T" piece	Coaxial
Laryngoscope	Straight blade	Straight blade	Child Macintosh	Child Macintosh	Adult Macintosh
Tracheal tubes (uncuffed)	2.5–3.5	3.5–4.0	4.0–5.0	5.0–6.0	5.5–7.0
Stylet	Small	Small	Small/medium	Medium	Medium
Suction catheter (FG)	6	8	10–12	14	14
Circulation:					
Intravenous cannula (G)	24/22	22	22/18	20/16	18/14
Central venous pressure cannula (G)	20	20	18	18	16
Arterial cannula (G)	24/22	22	22	22	20
Ancillary equipment:					
Nasogastric tube (FG)	8	10	10–12	12	12–14
Chest drain (CH)	10–14	12–18	14–20	14–24	16–30
Urinary catheter (CH)	5 G Feeding tube	5 G Feeding tube/ Foley (8)	Foley (8)	Foley (10)	Foley (10–12)
Cervical collar			Small	Small	Medium

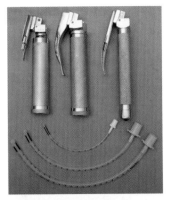

Laryngoscopes. (Left to right) Wisconsin, Sewerd, MacIntosh. With endotracheal tubes of various sizes for 0–10 years.

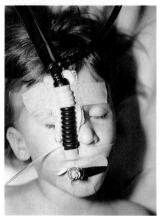

Correct fixation of Rees modified Ayres's "T" piece, endotracheal tube, and oral airway.

Artificial airway

If there is no gag reflex or if there is any doubt as to the adequacy of the airway an artificial airway is required. A Guedel airway should be inserted and the chin supported as described above. If assisting ventilation the lungs should be gently inflated with 100% oxygen with pressures of <20 cm H_2O. Higher pressures cause gaseous distension of the stomach, thus increasing the risk of regurgitation and resulting in diaphragmatic splinting.

Tracheal intubation

Orotracheal intubation should be performed when hypoxia has been reversed by ventilation with a mask. **Do not persistently attempt to intubate the trachea of a hypoxic child without giving oxygen beforehand with a mask and airway.**

Laryngoscopes with straight blades should be used for children younger than 1 year (with the epiglottis being raised on the posterior surface); curved blades are satisfactory in older children. As a rough guide a tube of similar external diameter to the child's small finger or nostril is appropriate. Uncuffed endotracheal tubes must be used for all children who have not reached puberty, and there should be a small leak of gas around the tube as the lungs are inflated. If there is no leak the tube should be exchanged for the next smaller size. The orotracheal tube should be positioned such that 2–5 cm of it (according to age) are below the vocal cords. The tube lengths recommended in the paediatric resuscitation chart should result in an appropriate position. Inadvertent endobronchial intubation is a potential hazard, and auscultation in the axillae for bilateral breath sounds is essential. Firm fixation of both tube and breathing circuit is vital.

Cricothyroidotomy

Needle cricothyroidotomy with a 14 G intravenous cannula is the preferred method of establishing airway access and control if bag and mask ventilation or intubation are unsuccessful. Tracheostomy should be undertaken only in controlled circumstances.

Gastric intubation

Acute gastric dilatation is commonly seen in the injured child. Almost all infants and children who are stressed swallow large quantities of air, and mask ventilation may add to this. Acute gastric dilatation may precipitate vomiting and aspiration, splint the diaphragm, and compress the inferior vena cava, diminishing venous return and thereby causing hypotension. A gastric tube must be passed in all injured children. If the cribriform plate is intact nasogastric intubation is the route of choice.

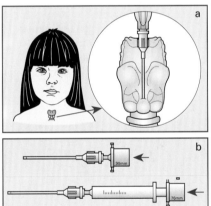
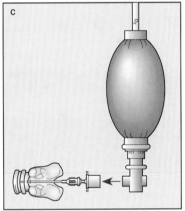

Technique for needle cricothyroidotomy. (a) The cricothyroid membrane is pierced at an angle of 45° by a 14 G cannula. Free aspiration of air confirms correct placement, and the cannula is advanced over the needle, which is then withdrawn; (b) a 3.0 mm endotracheal tube connector fits into the female end of the intravenous cannula or a 7.0 mm connector into the barrel of a 2 ml syringe; (c) the connector is attached to the oxygen circuit.

Breathing

Causes of inadequate ventilation

Bilateral
- Obstruction of upper respiratory tract
- Oesophageal intubation

Unilateral
- Pneumothorax
- Haemothorax
- Lung contusion
- Flail segment
- Bronchial rupture
- Foreign body in bronchus
- Rupture of diaphragm
- Endobronchial intubation

Ensure that both sides of the chest are being ventilated by inspection and auscultation. Look for central cyanosis and ensure that haemoglobin saturation measured with a pulse oximeter is above 90%. Count the respiratory rate, noting that normal values change with age.

Ventilation must be started if breathing is inadequate. Children who fail to respond to bag and mask ventilation will require intubation as will those who require therapeutic hyperventilation. Children should be ventilated at 15–20 breaths/minute, and infants 30–40 breaths/minute. Tidal volumes should be 10 ml/kg.

Circulation and control of bleeding

Normal values for paediatric vital signs in patients who are not crying

Age	Heart rate (beats/min)	Blood pressure (systolic) (mm Hg)	Respiratory rate (breaths/min)	Blood volume (ml/kg)
<1 year	120–140	70–90	30–40	90
2–5 years	100–120	80–90	20–30	80
5–12 years	80–100	90–110	15–20	80

As in any victim of trauma major external haemorrhage must be controlled by direct pressure. The pulse rate and blood pressure are then recorded, the capillary refill time estimated, and the peripheral skin temperature and colour noted. Normal values for vital signs vary with age.

Advanced trauma life support classification of shock in children

	Class I <15%	Class II 15%–25%	Class III 25%–40%	Class IV >40%
Cardiovascular system (heart rate in beats/min)	Heart rate ↑ 10–20% Blood pressure normal	Tachycardia (>150) Systolic blood pressure ↓ Pulse pressure ↓	Tachycardia (>150) Systolic blood pressure ↓↓ Pulse pressure ↓↓	Tachycardia/ bradycardia Severe hypotension Peripheral pulses absent
Respiratory rate (breaths/min)	Normal	Tachypnoea (35–40)	Tachypnoea	Respiratory rate falls
Skin	Normal	Cool, peripheries cool and clammy	Cold, clammy, cyanotic	Pale, cold
Central nervous system	Normal	Irritable, confused, aggressive	Lethargic	Comatose
Capillary refill time	Normal	Prolonged	Very prolonged	

A child's normal systolic blood pressure may be estimated by using the formula: blood pressure = 80 mm Hg + (2 × age). The increased physiological reserve of the child's circulation compared with that of adults means that vital signs may be only slightly abnormal despite considerable blood loss. Therefore the early diagnosis of impending shock in children is based on the appearance of the skin, the temperature of the extremities, the capillary refill time (normal <2 seconds), and altered sensorium. The degree of shock, and hence blood loss, can be estimated from the classification of shock. Fluid resuscitation should not be withheld until vital signs are abnormal.

Circulatory access

Venous access in hypovolaemic children with collapsed veins is difficult, especially in those less than 6 years old. Percutaneous cannulation of peripheral veins with an appropriately sized cannula should be attempted. In patients with appreciable abdominal injuries a vein draining to the superior vena cava should be chosen. If after two attempts access is not established the femoral or external jugular vein should be cannulated.

If all attempts at percutaneous cannulation fail a cut down should be undertaken over the median cephalic vein in the elbow or the long saphenous vein in the ankle.

In the interim intraosseous infusion is a useful method of emergency resuscitation in children. Crystalloids, colloids, and drugs can be given by this route, and the circulation time is usually less than 30 seconds. Fluids given by this route have to be infused under pressure, usually by syringe. Cellulitis or osteomyelitis are potential complications.

The sites for intraosseous infusion are:
(1) The anterior tibial plateau 3 cm below the tibial tuberosity.
(2) The inferior one third of femur 3 cm above the external condyle.

Enter perpendicular to the bone (using a 16 G or 18 G bone marrow needle). Marrow aspiration indicates correct positioning.

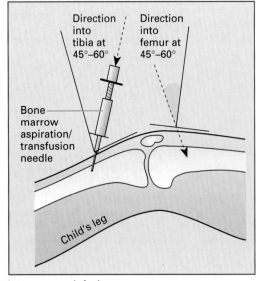

Intraosseous infusion.

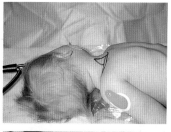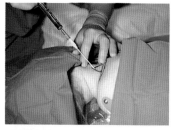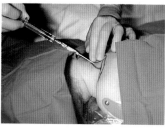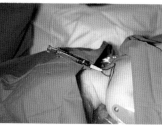

Cannulation of the right internal jugular vein. This should **never** be done if there is a suspicion of cervical spine injury.

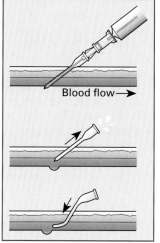

Transfix the vessel.

Blood flow→

Withdraw the needle then the cannula until blood flows freely

Advance the cannula into the vessel.

Technique for transfixion and cannulation of a peripheral artery.

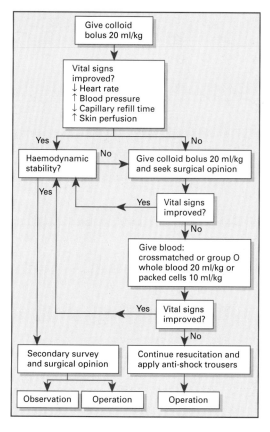

Having established venous access take blood samples for grouping and crossmatching, and measurement of full blood count, and urea and electrolyte concentrations.

Central venous cannulation in children is hazardous, especially if the patient is hypovolaemic, and should *never* be attempted by inexperienced doctors.

As in adults, a central venous pressure line is primarily for monitoring and not for giving fluids. Time must not be wasted inserting a central venous pressure line at the expense of other measures of basic life support during the initial resuscitation. Hypovolaemic children respond well to volume loading, allowing an adequate central venous pressure to be inferred from improvements in vital signs and skin perfusion.

When blood loss is massive (30%–40%), however, intravascular volume must be assessed with a central venous pressure line.

The series of four pictures shows the procedure for cannulation of the right internal jugular vein. Tilt the patient's head downwards; extend the neck with a sandbag under the shoulder (**there must be no suspicion of cervical spine injury**); turn the head to the left and identify the triangle formed by the clavicle—the base—and the two heads of sternocleidomastoid muscle (top left). With a strict aseptic technique pierce the skin at the apex of the triangle, aiming for the right nipple (top right). The internal jugular vein is very superficial and should be entered within 1–2 cm of the skin. Having punctured the vein, move the needle to a more horizontal position, then advance the cannula over the needle into the superior vena cava (bottom left). Withdraw the needle and ensure that blood can be aspirated freely (bottom right), then connect to a monitoring set.

Seriously injured patients should also have their intra-arterial pressure monitored. A transfixion technique is easiest in infants, and this should initially be attempted in the peripheral arteries.

Fluid administration

Initial resuscitation should be with colloid (Haemaccel, Gelofusine, hetastarch), or 4.5% albumin (human plasma protein fraction). All fluids must be warmed to body temperature. An initial dose of 20 ml/kg should be given as a bolus, after which the response should be assessed and the decision tree followed. Patients with class III or IV shock require blood. If necessary blood that is not crossmatched can be used; there is, however, usually time to get an immediate typed crossmatch that will eliminate serious reactions due to ABO incompatibility.

Whole blood, especially fresh whole blood, is rarely available. Red blood cells with a packed cell volume of 65%—75% are often supplied. Administration of blood with a high packed cell volume is difficult through the small (22 G or 24 G) cannulas used in infants. Reconstitution of packed cells to a normal packed cell volume with human plasma protein fraction (HPPF/albumin 4.5%) overcomes this problem but is time consuming.

Dysfunction and exposure

Glasgow Coma Scale (4–15 years)		Children's Coma Scale (<4 years)		
Response	Score	*Response*		Score
Eyes		Eyes		
Open spontaneously	4	Open spontaneously		4
Verbal command	3	React to speech		3
Pain	2	React to pain		2
No response	1	No response		1
Best motor response		Best motor response		
Verbal command:		Spontaneous or obeys verbal		
obeys	6	command		6
Painful stimulus:		*Painful stimulus:*		
Localises pain	5	Localises pain		
Flexion with pain	4	Withdraws in response to pain		4
		Abnormal flexion to pain		
Flexion abnormal	3	(decorticate posture)		3
Extension	2	(decerebrate posture)		2
No response	1	No response		1
Best verbal response		Best verbal response		
Orientated and converse	5	Smiles, orientated to sounds, follows objects, interacts		5
Disorientated and converse	4	*Crying* Consolable Inconsistently	*Interacts* Inappropriate	4
Inappropriate words	3	consolable	Moaning	3
Incomprehensible sounds	2	Inconsolable	Irritable	2
No response	1	No response	No response	1

SECONDARY SURVEY

Principles for the secondary survey

- Children should be assessed systematically according to a strict protocol
- Finding an injury should not stop the remainder of the evaluation
- Be gentle and pay particular attention to manipulation of the spinal cord axis
- Vital signs should be recorded repeatedly

Head and neck

Causes of secondary brain damage

Hypoxia
—Respiratory insufficiency

Cerebral ischaemia
—Systemic hypotension
—Fall in cerebral perfusion pressure secondary to raised intracranial pressure from cerebral oedema or an intracranial mass lesion

Ages at which acute subdural and extradural haematomas are usually seen in children and associated incidences of seizures and skull fractures

	Acute subdural haematomas	Extradural haematomas
Age at which usually seen	<12 months	>2 years
Associated incidence of seizures	High (75%)	Low (<25%)
Associated incidence of skull fractures	Low (30%)	High (75%)

Dysfunction

If the patient is old enough and well enough to cooperate the brain and spinal cord can be assessed rapidly by standard techniques. In young patients observation of motor function and ability to speak must suffice. An initial Glasgow coma scale score should be established. A rapid assessment should be made using the following simple scale: **A**lert, response to **V**oice, response to **P**ain, and **U**nresponsive. This should be followed by calculation of the first Glasgow Coma Scale Score.

Exposure

Removal of clothing is essential to allow adequate physical examination and facilitate practical procedures. Children, especially infants, however, lose heat rapidly as a result of their high ratio of surface area to weight, thin skin, and lack of subcutaneous tissue. Considerable heat loss may have occurred at the site of injury and during transportation. Monitoring temperature is a vital component of initial assessment. A fall in body temperature causes a rise in oxygen consumption as endogenous processes begin to increase heat production, peripheral vasoconstriction, and consequent lactic acidaemia. The ambient temperature of the resuscitation room should be raised and overhead heaters and warming blankets used. Plastic sheets can be used to cover exposed body parts.

After the primary survey, initial stabilisation of the cardiorespiratory system, and treatment of shock a complete physical examination takes place.

As in adult patients fully examine the head for lacerations; the skull for fractures; the eyes for injury (also remember penetrating injury) and pupillary function; the ears and nose for leakage of cerebrospinal fluid; the face for fractures and lacerations; the mouth for loose teeth; and, finally, the neck for cervical displacement. Frequent assessment of the Glasgow coma score is essential.

Primary brain damage that occurs at the time of the injury cannot be reversed. Secondary brain damage occurs as a result of cerebral hypoxia or ischaemia and can be minimised by maintaining oxygenation and an adequate cerebral perfusion pressure.

A child's brain is vulnerable to accelerative, decelerative, and shear forces which result in focal intracranial mass lesions (cerebral contusions, lacerations, and haemorrhages) and cerebral oedema. Raised intracranial pressure secondary to diffuse cerebral swelling is the most common cause of death in children with head injuries.

Acute subdural haematomas are often bilateral and are associated with a high incidence of seizures and a low incidence of skull fractures. If there is no history of appreciable trauma the possibility of non-accidental injury should be considered.

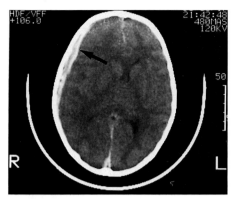

Computed tomogram showing right subdural haematoma.

Initial management of severe head injury

- Restoration of the circulating blood volume
- Tracheal intubation
- Adequate oxygenation (SaO$_2$ >90%)
- Hyperventilation (PaCO$_2$ 3.5–4.0 kPa)
- Administration of mannitol 0.5–1.0 g/kg

Criteria for skull radiography after head injury in children

- Age <1 year
- Loss of consciousness ≥5 minutes
- Lethargy, coma, or stupor
- Focal neurological signs
- Skull penetration
- Skull depression
- Palpable scalp haematoma
- Cerebrospinal fluid from nose or ear
- Blood in middle ear
- Battle's sign
- Racoon eyes

Extradural haematomas are most often unilateral and associated with a high incidence of skull fractures and a low incidence of seizures. The biphasic presentation of extradural haematomas ("lucid interval") is less common in children.

About 75% of skull fractures are linear, but they may be depressed, compound, or basal, and in children of less than 3 years, the cranial sutures can undergo traumatic separation (diasteal fractures).

The clinical manifestations of raised intracranial pressure or skull fractures are the same in children as in adults. Infants with open fontanelles and mobile sutures, however, are more tolerant to an expanding intracranial mass, although when decompensation does occur it is rapid and often irrecoverable. A bulging fontanelle or suture diastases in an infant implies serious cerebral trauma.

As in adults an initial Glasgow coma score of <7 or a declining score are indications for immediate aggressive management. In particular, restoration of the circulating volume is vital and should not be limited by considerations of fluid restriction to control cerebral oedema. A neurosurgical opinion should be sought urgently, and if the patient is haemodynamically stable computed tomography should be performed immediately. Intracranial pressure monitoring should be considered early.

In children, head injury alone does not usually produce shock and hypotension due to hypovolaemia; most bleeding usually occurs elsewhere in the body. Extensive scalp lacerations, however, may bleed sufficiently to cause hypovolaemic shock, and in small infants intracranial haemorrhage may be enough to cause hypovolaemia.

After head injury vomiting and seizures are more common in children than in adults. Both symptoms tend to be self limiting, but if either persists a serious head injury should be suspected. Repeated seizures cause an increase in intracranial pressure by increasing cerebral blood flow, and anticonvulsants should be given. Intravenous diazepam 0.15–0.25 mg/kg is the drug of first choice; this may cause respiratory depression, so be prepared to provide artificial ventilation. Follow this with phenytoin 15–20 mg/kg by slow intravenous injection (1–2 mg/kg/min); monitor the electrocardiogram continuously during the injection.

Minor head injury is extremely common in children; the overwhelming majority of children with such injury do not develop intracranial pathology and the need for radiography is often questionable.

Neck and spine

Confusing radiological features of children's cervical spines

Growth centres resemble fractures
- Cartilaginous plate at the base of the odontoid (closes at between 3 and 5 years)
- Secondary ossification centre at apex of odontoid (present from 2–12 years)
- Secondary ossification centre at tip of spinous processes

Pseudosubluxation
- Anterior displacement of C2 on C3 (30% of children <7 years). Much less commonly C3 on C4. Perform radiography in neutral and extension positions if clinically safe

Hypermobility
- Increased distance between dens and anterior arch of C1 (15% of children <5 years)

Spinal cord injuries are rare in children, constituting only 5% of all spinal cord trauma. But there should be a high index of suspicion in any child with major trauma, especially if he or she has an appreciable head injury.

Careful clinical and radiological examination should be undertaken (see chapter 8). Assessing paralysis and altered sensation, however, can be very difficult, especially in infants. Mass flexion withdrawal in response to stimulation may be indistinguishable from normal withdrawal in this age group. Furthermore, 50% of children with serious spinal injuries have normal radiographs, and radiological normality should not deter a clinical diagnosis of spinal injury. Conversely, there are several peculiarities in radiographs of the immature spine that may lead to overdiagnosis of spinal injury.

Paediatric trauma

Thorax

> **Occult chest injuries in children**
>
> - Pulmonary contusion
> - Pulmonary laceration
> - Intrapulmonary haemorrhage
> - Tracheobronchial tear
> - Myocardial contusion
> - Diaphragmatic rupture
> - Partial aortic or other great vessel disruption
> - Oesophageal tears

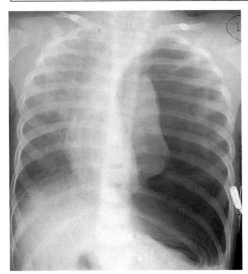

Radiograph of left tension pneumothorax causing deviation of the mediastinum to the right.

> **Indications for cardiothoracic referral:**
>
> - Continuing air leak or haemorrhage after insertion of chest drain
> - Cardiac tamponade
> - Disruption of great vessels

Abdomen

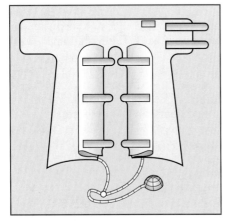

Pneumatic antishock trousers will maintain central circulating volume during fluid resuscitation.

Blunt chest trauma is common in children whereas penetrating injury is rare; but the approach to diagnosis and management is the same as in adults. About 15%–20% of children with major injuries have chest trauma that requires immediate management. Early diagnosis is essential: of the children who die of chest injury more than 90% die in the first few hours after the accident. The vast majority of thoracic injuries (85%–90%) can be managed by standard procedures. Remember that patients with thoracic trauma have a high incidence of associated injuries (>50%), most commonly of the head, abdomen, or an extremity.

The chest wall should be examined for bruising, wounds, and asymmetry of movement. The high compliance of a child's chest wall, however, allows ready transfer of energy to intrathoracic structures, and appreciable organ damage may be present with minimal evidence of chest wall injury.

The mobility of mediastinal structures in children means that cardiovascular and ventilatory compromise occur readily as a result of trauma causing mediastinal shift.

If a pneumothorax (indicated by inequality of air entry) is under tension it requires immediate drainage. Open pneumothorax is unusual in children. Flail segments are also uncommon in children but require early treatment with chest drainage, intermittent positive pressure ventilation and positive end expiratory pressure. Haemoptysis, subcutaneous emphysema, and a persistent air leak after drainage of a pneumothorax all suggest underlying lung damage.

Patients with pulmonary contusion present with tachypnoea, breathlessness, and hypoxia. The symptoms are often exacerbated by inhalation of gastric contents, especially if the abdomen has been compressed. If the child has undergone a garrotting injury tracheal rupture should be suspected, especially if there is subcutaneous emphysema in the neck. Noisy breathing and a persistent leak through the chest drain suggest a tracheal or major bronchial tear. As in adults diaphragmatic rupture, most commonly on the left side, is often missed clinically but should be suspected if the left side of the diaphragm is not clearly visualised in the chest radiograph.

Myocardial contusion is rare in children but is suggested by arrhythmias in a child who has sustained blunt trauma to the anterior chest wall. Continuous electrocardiography is vital. Cardiac tamponade due to haemopericardium is also rare because penetrating injury is unusual in children. The signs are the same as in adults, and drainage using a 14 G intravenous cannula should be by the left subxiphoid route. Although mediastinal mobility in children means that there is a lower incidence of rupture of the great vessels compared with adults, aortic rupture (which is most common at the origin of the left subclavian artery) is suggested by a widened mediastinum, fractures of the first or second ribs, and obliteration of the aortic knuckle in the chest radiograph.

Clinical assessment of the signs of hypovolaemic shock should be frequently repeated to assess the response to fluid resuscitation.

The basic principle governing the evaluation of a child with a possible abdominal injury is to determine whether an operation is necessary either for an acute abdomen or for controlling haemorrhage.

As in thoracic injuries blunt trauma is most common. Penetrating wounds are rare but, when present, require an operation. If haemorrhage is substantial and rapid the use of pneumatic antishock trousers may be life saving, providing time for resuscitation and exploring the abdomen.

Early passage of a nasogastric tube of appropriate size is essential in children. Careful and gentle clinical examination of the conscious child will produce evidence of appreciable abdominal injury, which may be present despite minimal indications of trauma in the abdominal wall. The pattern and methods of clinical examination are the same as in adults.

As in adults the spleen and liver are the most commonly injured solid organs, but rapid deceleration forces cause abdominal compression and may result in other injuries. A renal injury should be suspected in every child with tenderness of the flank and red blood cells in the urine. The lumbar spine, ribs, and pelvis are also commonly injured.

Assessment of the abdomen may be difficult in an unconscious child. Haemodynamic instability or questionable abdominal findings are indications for computed tomography. Also, if the patient receives general anaesthesia for other surgery, lavage can help to determine whether abdominal exploration is required. A paediatric size peritoneal dialysis catheter is inserted through the lower abdominal midline under direct vision, remembering that a child's abdominal wall is much thinner than an adult's. Then 10 ml/kg of Ringer-lactate solution is run in over 10 minutes. Lavage results in peritoneal irritation for up to 48 hours, making subsequent assessment difficult. In practice it is much less often needed in children than in adults and a decision to perform lavage should not be undertaken lightly.

The rate of urine output must be measured through a catheter in children with trauma, unless they can void spontaneously. The approach (through the urethra or suprapubic) is determined by the clinical evidence of urethral injury. Urine should always be dipstick tested for blood, glucose, etc.

All children with multiple injuries should undergo cervical spine, chest, and pelvic radiography. If damage to the urinary tract is suspected a one shot intravenous pyelogram in the resuscitation room can often provide useful information in patients who require urgent abdominal exploration. Many North American centres advocate thoracic and abdominal computed tomography for investigating children with multiple injuries, provided that they are haemodynamically stable.

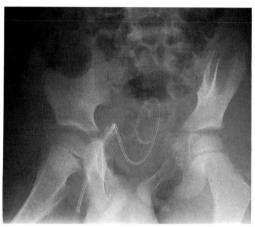

Radiograph showing fractured pelvis caused by a crush injury. A suprapubic catheter is in situ.

Skeletal and soft tissue injuries

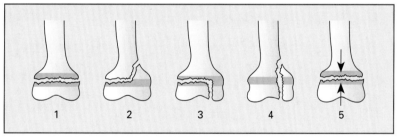

The Salter-Harris classification of epiphyseal fractures.

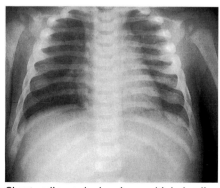

Chest radiograph showing multiple healing rib fractures after non-accidental injury.

The principles of management of skeletal and soft tissue damage are the same as those for adults. In children the history of the injury is important. The radiological diagnosis of skeletal injury around the joints is more difficult in children because of the growth plate and lack of mineralisation of the epiphysis. Radiographs of the opposite side (if uninjured) may be helpful.

The pattern of fractures is different in children. They may be through the growth plate (Salter-Harris classification[1] types I-V), greenstick (only through one cortex of a long bone), or buckle (bony angulation without a fracture). Because of potential arresting of growth, malalignment of joints, and traumatic arthritis it is important to recognise fractures through the epiphysis. Supracondylar fractures at the elbow have a high incidence of associated vascular injury. The proportional blood loss after pelvic or long bone fractures in children is greater and may be an important cause of initial haemodynamic instability. Old healed fractures should alert the medical team to the possibility of non-accidental injury.

Burns

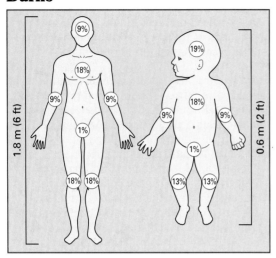

Scalds from hot water are the most common cause of burns in children, and management does not differ appreciably from that of adult patients (see chapter on burns). The change in body proportions as children grow means that calculation of the percentage total body surface area burnt cannot be based on the adult "rule of nines". Accurate estimation of the percentage of the total body surface area burnt requires the use of detailed charts.[2]

Non-accidental injury

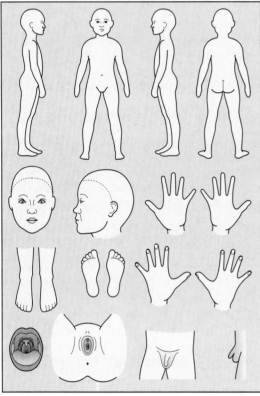

Diagram used for precise marking of injuries in a suspected case of non-accidental injury.

A wide variety of injuries can be caused by physical child abuse. Various points in the history and examination should suggest the possibility of non-accidental injury. Initial resuscitation and management of the battered child are the prime responsibilities of the casualty medical team, but the need to inform the appropriate authorities must not be overlooked. Careful recording of injuries is vital, and standard diagrams should be available for this purpose.

Diagnostic criteria for non-accidental injury

- Delay in seeking medical advice
- Account of the accident is vague and inconsistent among parties
- Discrepancy between the history and the degree of injury
- Parental behaviour is abnormal, lack of concern for their child
- Interaction between child and parents is abnormal
- Finger tip bruising, especially over upper arms, trunk, sides of face, ears, or neck
- Bizarre injuries—for example, bites, cigarette burns, or rope marks
- Sharply demarcated burns in unusual areas
- Perioral injuries—for example, torn frenulum
- Retinal haemorrhage
- Multiple subdural haemorrhages
- Ruptured internal organs without a history of major trauma
- Perianal or genital injury
- Long bone fractures in children <3 years
- Previous injuries—for example, old scars, healing fractures

---

Pain relief

Patients with appreciable head injuries whose conscious level is depressed or fluctuating should not receive opioid analgesics.

Control of pain

- After resuscitation give morphine 50 μg/kg intravenously
- Titrate further doses of 25 μg/kg against patient's response
- Do not give narcotic drugs to patients with head injuries

Adequate control of pain is humane and will improve a child's cooperation with diagnosis, investigation, and management. After initial fluid resuscitation a bolus of 50 μg/kg of morphine should be given intravenously. Further doses may be given at 10 minute intervals, titrated against the patient's response to just control pain.

Throughout the secondary survey the child's response to resuscitation and general condition should be constantly reassessed. Subsequent management depends on the expertise and facilities of the receiving hospital. If the anaesthetic, surgical, and intensive care services are not suited to children a protocol for transfer to a designated paediatric centre should be an important part of the initial evaluation and management.

1 Salter RB, Harris WR. Injuries involving the epiphyseal plate. *American Journal of Bone and Joint Surgery* 1963; **45**: 587–622.
2 Lund CC, Bowder NC. The estimation of area of burns. *Surg Gynecol Obstet* 1944; **79**: 353–60.

The paediatric resuscitation chart is by P A Oakley and was devised from the guidelines of the Resuscitation Council (UK). The radiographs were kindly provided by Drs B Kendall, D Shaw, C Hall, and D Hatch, Hospital for Sick Children, Great Ormond Street, London.

19 TRAUMA IN THE ELDERLY

Carl L Gwinnutt, Michael A Horan

It has been estimated that in the USA elderly people account for about one third of the cost of all trauma care

Old people are seriously injured less often than any other sector of the population but mortality and morbidity are higher than in any other age group, regardless of the severity of the injury. Fewer injuries are associated with motor vehicle accidents, falls being the main cause. This is because of changes in vision, vestibular function, proprioception, prolonged motor reaction time, and neurological and musculoskeletal diseases.

Life expectancy of men and women at different ages

Age (years)	Active life expectancy Men	Women	Dependent life expectancy Men	Women
65	9.5	10.5	4.5	9.0
75	6.5	3.0	7.0	6.5
85	3.0	3.0	2.5	5.0

Until recently, the outcome of trauma care for elderly people was poor but it is rapidly becoming clear that early and aggressive therapeutic intervention accompanied by invasive monitoring can considerably improve it. Age alone accounts for little of the variance in outcome in patients in intensive care units; it is the underlying (patho)physiology that is the main determinant. It is therefore of great importance to detect and correct physiological and metabolic derangements which accompany major trauma to maximise survival.

Primary survey and resuscitation

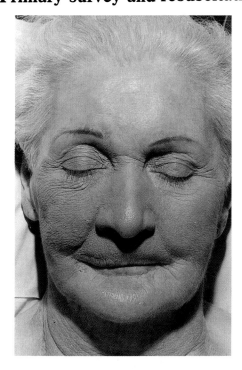

Airway management with protection of the cervical spine

Many older patients are edentulous but some are not and may have loose, inconveniently situated, or carious teeth. Furthermore, resorption of the mandible and lax cheeks may make maintenance of the airway more difficult.

Well fitting dentures may be left in place initially, but the doctor dealing with the airway should record this and inform the team leader. If dentures are removed, they must be inspected to ensure they are complete, particularly if they have been fractured. Airway adjuncts must be used with care because the soft tissues of the oropharynx and nasopharynx are more prone to damage, particularly the turbinates which may bleed profusely.

Intubation is generally straightforward, but beware of temporomandibular arthritis which may limit mouth opening. During all the manoeuvres to establish and maintain a patent airway, great care must be taken with the cervical spine because arthritis (osteoarthritis and rheumatoid disease) is the rule rather than the exception. Consequently, these trauma patients are particularly prone to cervical cord or nerve injury if subjected to excessive flexion or extension of the neck.

Trauma in the elderly

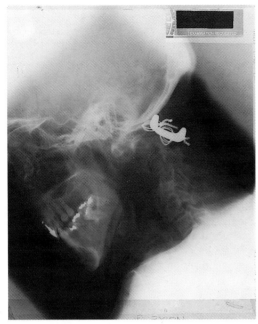

Lateral radiograph of cervical spine showing severe degenerative changes.

> **All patients should be given 100% oxygen initially, regardless of whether they have chronic lung disease or carbon dioxide retention.** It is the partial pressure of oxygen in arterial blood (PaO_2) that is maintaining respiratory drive, not the inspired oxygen concentration

Aging and incidence of ischaemic heart disease (annual rate/1000)

Age group (years)	Men	Women
35–44	5	1
45–54	11	4
55–64	19	10
65–74	23	14
75–84	30	22
85–94	39	41

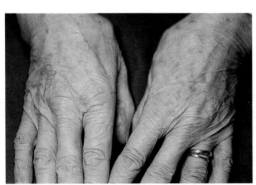

Intravenous access to the circulation may be difficult, particularly in patients with diabetes, obesity, and connective tissue disorders.

Breathing

Lung function in older patients is affected by changes in the chest wall, ventilatory muscles, and lung parenchyma. The thorax becomes stiffer as a result of calcification of the costal cartilages, reduction in the intervertebral disc spaces, and coexisting crush fractures of the vertebral bodies. Together, these produce an increase in the anteroposterior diameter of the chest and reduced rib excursion. The elastic recoil properties of the lung also decrease with age, which reduces the ease of ventilation and decreases compliance. In addition, there is an increase in the collapse of small airways during expiration, leading to non-uniform ventilation and air trapping. Collectively, these cause a small reduction in PaO_2. These changes, together with an impaired mucociliary escalator, predispose elderly patients to atelectasis, pneumonia, and hypoventilation.

For the reasons given above, it is often difficult to support ventilation with oxygen given by facemask and hypoxia can develop rapidly. If there is any doubt about the adequacy of oxygenation, mechanical ventilation with 100% oxygen should be started early. Pneumothoraces are produced more commonly in this age group, particularly in those patients with chronic lung diseases, and the team leader should be constantly aware of this. Frequent inspection of the chest for symmetry of movement, the development of surgical emphysema, and equality of breath sounds, will ensure rapid recognition of this complication. Arterial blood gas analysis should be done as soon as possible to ensure the adequacy of oxygenation and ventilation. In view of the serious potential problems that may arise in these patients, the help of an anaesthetist should be sought early.

Circulation and control of haemorrhage

The incidence of ischaemic heart disease increases with age but its prevalence in old age is unknown. Necropsy studies suggest a prevalence in those over 65 of about 60%, but in the living of similar age estimates vary between 10% and 30%.

Even in healthy people, advancing age is associated with cardiovascular changes. Increased stiffness of the arterial walls leads to an increase in systolic blood pressure and left ventricular hypertrophy. Resting cardiac output is maintained, but the ability to mount a compensatory tachycardia is reduced. Healthy old people compensate by increased venous return and raise cardiac output predominantly through the Starling mechanism, so a reduced intravascular volume may lead to a rapid reduction in cardiac output.

The initial fluid for resuscitation is warmed Ringer's lactate, but the response must be continuously monitored accurately because of the reduced tolerance of either hypovolaemia or fluid overload. It is important to remember that measurements of pulse and blood pressure give only limited information about intravascular volume. This is particularly true in patients with heart disease, indwelling pacemakers, and those taking cardiovascular drugs. Early consideration should be given to invasive monitoring (for example, central venous pressure, pulmonary artery wedge pressure, and cardiac output). Central venous pressure measurements may be misleading in those with heart disease and expert advice should be sought early.

The urinary bladder should be catheterised to measure urine output, and a strict aseptic technique must be ensured. Aging is usually associated with loss of renal cortical structures, a fall in the glomerular filtration rate, and decline in renal function by about 1 ml/min for each year after the age of 40 years. These changes make old people particularly vulnerable to incompetent fluid and metabolic management.

Cardiac dysrhythmias and conduction abnormalities are common, even in apparently healthy old people. Adequate oxygenation should be ensured and cardiac contusions excluded before they are discounted.

ECG abnormalities in apparently healthy old people

- Atrial ectopics
- Ventricular ectopics
- Atrial fibrillation
- Left anterior hemiblock
- First degree heart block

Confusion is a common symptom in acutely ill old people. In its evaluation, consider withdrawal of psychotropic drugs (particularly benzodiazepines), and alcohol

Dysfunction of the central nervous system

Most confused, ill, old people are not demented. Confusion can be a feature of almost any illness in the aged—particularly infection, fluid and metabolic derangements, head injury, and as a result of medicines or their withdrawal. In addition, multiple sensory impairments may lead to disorientation and inappropriate responses and make assessment difficult.

Initial treatment is to ensure adequate cerebral perfusion with oxygenated blood rather than to assume that this is the patient's normal mental state. In unconscious elderly patients, consider intracerebral haemorrhage as both the cause and effect of coexisting trauma.

Exposure

All patients must be completely undressed to ensure that all injuries are identified. It is, however, important to prevent the development or worsening of hypothermia. As soon as the examination is completed, the patient should be wrapped in blankets. Core temperature measurements are essential and one should not rely on simply feeling the patient's peripheries to estimate body temperature.

Secondary survey

Injuries arise from the transfer of energy at rates and in amounts that exceed the tolerance of tissues. In old people, particularly old women, bone strength may be appreciably reduced and fractures may occur after only modest transfers of energy. Age-related changes in other organs and tissues make them particularly vulnerable to injury, so a head-to-toe examination must be undertaken after even apparently minor injuries. This will also ensure the detection of coincidental medical problems and the institution of appropriate treatment.

During physical examination care should be taken to maintain the usual anatomical position for the particular patient. It is particularly important to avoid producing traction and compression neuropathies (especially in the operating room) that may compromise rehabilitation. Extreme vigilance must be exercised during "log rolling", particularly if the patient is unconscious. The age-related changes described above make such patients vulnerable to iatrogenic damage to the cervical cord or nerve roots.

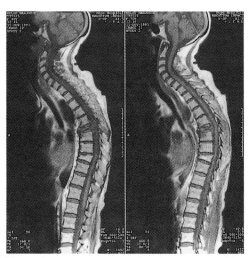

Magnetic resonance scan showing osteoporotic spine with collapse of T6 and T9.

Consideration must also be given to the prevention of decubitus ulcers. Appropriate pressure-dispersing surfaces should be readily available and all patients with multiple injuries must be considered to be at high risk. Consequently, prevention must begin in the emergency department. Initial x ray examinations should include the standard three films of the cervical spine, chest, and pelvis. The presence of coexisting medical illness and disease of bone and joints may make interpretation difficult, and the advice of more experienced colleagues should be sought early.

Nerves at particular risk from compression or traction

- Axillary nerve
- Radial nerve (in the spiral groove)
- Common peroneal nerve

Head injuries

As the brain ages, its dura becomes tightly adherent to the skull which makes epidural haematomas uncommon. A progressive loss of brain volume leads to an increase in the space around the brain that is thought to protect it from contusions, but makes subdural haematomas more likely. Even mild head injuries particularly in patients with pre-existing cognitive impairment, may lead to permanent neurological damage. If there is a skull fracture and an associated hemiparesis, a traumatic intracranial haematoma should be assumed and not a stroke. Similarly, confusion lasting more than 12 hours after head injury, even in a patient with no skull fracture, is an indication for a computed tomogram (CT). Any deterioration demands immediate action. CT should be done in all patients who are unconscious for more than five minutes after a head injury.

The outcome is extremely poor in elderly patients who have sustained head injuries sufficient to cause immediate coma that persists after hypoxia and hypovolaemia have been corrected. Neurosurgical intervention is not warranted for most of these patients.

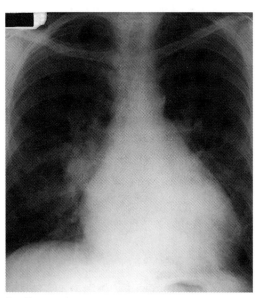

Cardiomegaly

Allergies
Medication
Past medical history
Last meal
Events leading to the injury

Chest trauma

Rib fractures often complicate even mild blunt trauma to the chest in old people. Such fractures heal slowly and are often poorly tolerated. These patients must be watched carefully and the need for mechanical ventilation frequently reassessed. Those with more severe blunt chest trauma, such as those with penetrating injuries, are managed in the same way as younger patients.

Abdominal trauma

The principles of care for elderly patients with abdominal trauma follow those already outlined in Chapter 9, but it must be remembered that old people are intolerant of both shock and unnecessary laparotomy. Their assessment therefore demands a sense of urgency and a high degree of clinical acumen.

Those who have a history or clinical evidence of previous major abdominal surgery should have either CT or an ultrasound scan of the abdomen rather than diagnostic peritoneal lavage.

Fractures

In old people with multiple injuries, fractures must be stabilised to permit optimal positioning and movement, both for immediate management and later rehabilitation. While isolated fractures of the humeral shaft are managed conservatively, there is no logic to such management in a patient with leg injuries who will need to use a walking frame or crutches for mobilisation. The aim of treatment should be to undertake the least invasive, most definitive, procedure with a view to early mobilisation as soon as other problems permit. Prolonged inactivity and disuse may seriously limit the eventual functional outcome.

AMPLE

A detailed history is particularly important and no source of information should be overlooked. The ambulance personnel will be able to give details of the immediate event and, when it occurred in the patient's home, may have brought medications with them. One member of the team should try to obtain hospital records and contact the general practitioner to find out about illnesses and medicines which may influence future management (see Chapter 12). Sometimes the patient may be able to give information directly while those with diabetes, on anticoagulants, or on steroid hormones, may be carrying a medication card.

Communicating with deaf patients may be particularly difficult. Check that any hearing aid is working and switched on. Shouting tends to use high frequency sounds and may be counterproductive in patients with presbyacusis. The voice should be lowered and the patient, wearing spectacles if needed, should be in a position to watch the speaker's lips. Significant confusion can usually be assessed by checking that the patient knows where they are, what day it is, and why they were brought to hospital. However, remember that even people who are not confused may not be able to cooperate because of pain and anxiety.

Conclusion

The photograph on p 107 is reproduced with the patient's permission.

Elderly patients have a particularly high mortality and are extremely vulnerable to less than optimal management. A system of trauma care must be prepared to cope with this group of patients and their special needs. The trauma team must be aware of the anatomical and physiological changes that accompany aging and how these factors, together with the effects of coexisting illnesses and medications, make special demands on their skills. Oversights and thoughtlessness in initial management of patients may have serious adverse consequences on recovery and eventual hospital discharge.

Elderly patients should be informed of what is happening and, where possible, be encouraged to participate in treatment decisions. Not all old people are demented. This does not mean they should necessarily receive identical treatment to younger people; instead, they must be managed in a way that is appropriate to their needs in the light of the likely outcome.

20 PREHOSPITAL CARE

Carl L Gwinnutt, Alastair W Wilson, Peter Driscoll

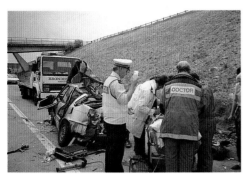
Scene of crash.

The principles of resuscitation are the same in the prehospital phase as in hospital, but the clinician is faced by greater impediments to success. Prehospital care may have been started by bystanders with a variable knowledge of first aid and continued by ambulance service personnel or paramedics, each of whom has a range of clinical skills and experience. Whatever the level of skills of those involved, the public will accord members of the emergency services with unwarranted abilities. The hostility of the environment and the stress of working in unfamiliar surroundings, often with inquisitive and intrusive onlookers, should not be underestimated.

On arrival at the scene

The three tiers of safety

- Yourself
- The scene
- The patients

Safety

All accident sites are dangerous. At road traffic accidents, for example, passing drivers may be distracted and cause secondary accidents by shunting cars in front; they may take a short cut on the hard shoulder, thereby endangering the rescuers. Training, appropriate clothing, the correct equipment, and common sense, are therefore required by helpers at accident sites.

Personal safety begins with immunisation against tetanus and hepatitis. On arrival at the incident, if the emergency services are present, report to the ambulance incident officer, who will tell you about the type of incident, whether the scene has been declared safe by the police and fire services, and how you can best help. You will be prevented from approaching the scene if you are inappropriately dressed or the environment is still unsafe. Protective, visible clothing is therefore essential. Furthermore, when moving about accident sites beware of jagged metal edges, glass, extrication equipment, rubble, and blood. Constant vigilance is required so that the risks of fire, sudden movement of heavy objects, electricity, or cables snapping under tension, may be identified.

Minimum clothing requirements

- Warm underclothing
- Fire-retardant suit with reflective bands
- High visibility jacket marked DOCTOR or NURSE
- Hard hat, with visor, goggles, and head-light
- Water and oil resistant footwear
- Latex gloves, for patient contact
- Ear defenders
- Heavy duty gloves (Firecraft type) for protection

Reading the scene

Observation of the accident scene, and analysis of the cause of the incident and the nature of damage to vehicles will give valuable clues as to the type of injuries victims may have sustained. An overall view will provide details of the number and type of vehicles involved, speed, direction of impact, and whether a vehicle has rolled over. The nature of the accident and an inspection of the interior of the vehicles for the degree of intrusion, position of occupants, and use of seatbelts, will also convey an idea of the likely injuries. Although mechanism of injury is only 25% specific for serious injury it should be part of the report that is given to the hospital with the patient. Polaroid photography of the scene greatly helps in providing this information.

Indications for transportation to a hospital able to receive patients with major trauma

- Penetrating injury to the chest, abdomen, head, neck, or groin
- Two or more proximal long bone fractures
- Burns covering >15% of body area or burns to the face or airway
- Evidence of high energy impact
  Falls of ≥6 m (≥20 ft)
  Crash speed of ≥32 km/h (≥20 mph)
  Inward deformity of the car of 0·6 m (2 ft)
  Rearward displacement of the front axle
  Intrusion of the passenger compartment of 38 cm (15 in) on the
    patient's side or 50 cm (20 in) on opposite side
  Ejection of the patient
  Rollover
  Death of a car occupant
  Pedestrian hit at ≥32 km/h (≥20 mph)
  Abnormal values for physiological variables

Primary survey and resuscitation

All personnel involved in prehospital care must be familiar with their equipment. It should be checked daily for completeness and function and to ensure familiarity. Resuscitation is conducted using the ABCDE principles, but, the patient's injuries and response to resuscitation will often preclude completion of the primary survey before transportation.

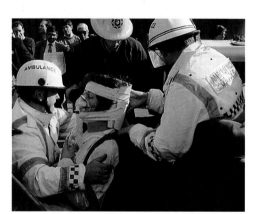

Cervical collar.

Airway and cervical spine control

Complete familiarity and competence with airway skills is essential for all personnel involved in prehospital care. Reduced levels of consciousness with positional airway obstruction are common and require urgent attention. Vomit and facial injuries may complicate management. If the patient is unable to maintain an airway it should be created and secured. This may mean using simple techniques initially because of lack of access. Tracheal intubation is often difficult and drugs should not be used to facilitate this unless the doctor is also competent at creating an airway surgically. The prehospital environment is not the place to learn these skills.

High concentrations of oxygen are given through a reservoir mask, bag-valve-mask, or ventilator. The cervical and axial spine must be protected by manual immobilisation and this is best achieved with help from emergency personnel. A rigid collar provides limited immobilisation which can be augmented with an extrication device or back board. Beware of taping the patient's head to a back board without securing the torso, as any movement of the patient on the board can result in the neck twisting.

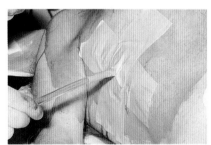

Chest drain in place.

Breathing

Underlying injury is often diagnosed by using tactile and visual observations. Breathing rates of less than 9 breaths/minute are always abnormal, but in the upper range rates of over 25 breaths/minute should also give cause for concern. Tracheal position, symmetry of movement, and pain may be the only clues to an underlying lung and chest wall injury. Changes in percussion note may not be audible but may be felt. Surrounding noise often makes breath sounds impossible to assess by auscultation.

Inadequate ventilation despite a patent airway requires ventilatory support. Initially this may be achieved using a bag-valve-mask technique until the trachea can be intubated.

If a clinical diagnosis of tension pneumothorax is made it should be treated immediately by needle thoracocentesis. Haemothoraces and pneumothoraces must be drained, particularly if positive pressure ventilation is to be instituted (see chapter 4).

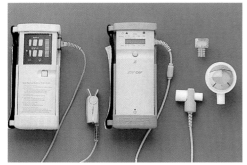

Pulse oximeter and infrared and chemical end tidal CO$_2$ analysers.

Patients with severe head injuries require early mechanical ventilation to avoid hypercarbia and the consequent rise in intracranial pressure (see chapter 6).

Pulse oximetry is a useful guide to oxygenation, provided that the peripheral circulation is adequate. The efficacy of ventilation can be further monitored by end tidal carbon dioxide measurement, using either infrared analysers or simple chemical indicators.

Circulation with control of haemorrhage

If bleeding is visible and controllable, apply external pressure. Optimally, two large bore cannulas should then be inserted and an adequate volume of fluid given (see chapter 5). Avoid placing them in veins directly over unsplinted joints or distal to fractures, and ensure that they are secure. If extrication is likely to be prolonged, a blood sample, clearly marked, should be taken and sent ahead to the receiving hospital for crossmatching.

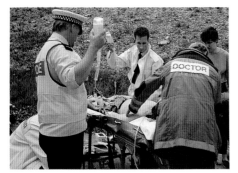

Crash victim with two intravenous lines.

If possible, all intravenous fluids should be warmed, particularly in winter. If the patient is erect and trapped, even greater volumes of intravenous fluids will be required to maintain venous return. Pulse and blood pressure must be monitored and recorded at regular intervals and the ECG displayed and recorded as necessary.

Dysfunction

The Glasgow coma scale score and response of the pupils to light should be noted. If the patient is conscious, an assessment of spinal cord function can be made by asking the patient to move fingers or feet. If there is any doubt, however, it is safer to assume that there is a spinal injury and immobilise the back accordingly.

Exposure

Exposure may cause injured patients to become hypothermic, particularly in wet and windy conditions or when they are trapped. Enough exposure to allow assessment and treatment of life threatening and debilitating injuries before extraction is required. Once this is achieved, the patient must be covered and kept warm and dry.

Problems at the accident site

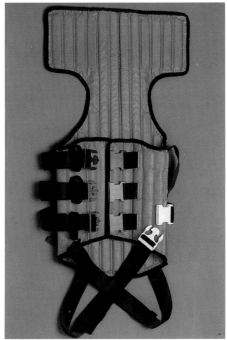

Kendrick extraction device.

Entrapment

Entrapment hinders resuscitation and the management of injuries. The fire service is responsible for extraction but it is important that there is close coordination of activity with the medical services to ensure the patient's safety. Doctors undertaking prehospital care must therefore have an understanding of extrication techniques.

Throughout extraction ensure the ABCs are managed and protect endotracheal tubes, intravenous access, and monitoring equipment. The patient must also be shielded from the effects of cutting equipment, broken glass, and impinging bodywork. Protect the fire service from medical "sharps". Adequate intravenous access is essential before the release of compressed limbs which may precipitate acute haemorrhage and hypovolaemia.

In unconscious patients, or those in whom the mechanism of injury suggests spinal cord damage, adequate immobilisation is essential. Rigid collars (for example, Stifneck, Vertebrace) help, but only partially stabilise the cervical spine. A spinal immobilisation device (Kendrick Extraction Device (KED) or Russell Extraction Device (RED)) should therefore be used to improve immobilisation, but these may be slow to apply and difficult to remove. Occasionally, a long spine board may be slid under the patient's back once the seat back has been removed, to facilitate extraction.

Before the patient is moved, give a warning about what is about to happen. Ensure that intravenous lines remain secure and that the endotracheal tube is disconnected during extraction and reconnected again afterwards. If the patient is to be monitored properly, the doctor must not be involved with lifting.

Analgesia

Adequate analgesia is important in injured, trapped patients. Entonox (50% oxygen and 50% nitrous oxide) is of limited use for short procedures in patients who are breathing spontaneously. It has to be given without interruption, otherwise its analgesic action is lost. It must not be used in patients who are at risk of pneumothorax or if there is clinical evidence of a fractured base of skull.

Opiates (morphine or diamorphine) can be diluted and given intravenously together with an antiemetic, and the dose titrated against response. Local anaesthetic techniques, such as femoral nerve block for fractured femurs or intercostal blocks for fractured ribs, are of value, particularly if the patient faces a long journey to hospital.

If there is no sign of head injury, subanaesthetic or anaesthetic doses of ketamine will provide good analgesia to facilitate extrication, but some patients experience terrifying hallucinations during recovery from this agent which may cause problems later—for example, during transport to hospital.

Anaesthesia is commonly required to allow tracheal intubation before a patient becomes deeply unconscious or to prevent a rise in intracranial pressure in a patient with a head injury. The same techniques are used as in the hospital but particular attention must be paid to restoring circulating volume adequately before induction, because of the vasodilating and cardiac depressant effects of anaesthetics. Remember also that muscle relaxants reduce the patient's ability to splint fractures and that the axial skeleton is particularly at risk.

Records

Accurate written records of all procedures and response to treatment must be noted on a prehospital care chart. Vital signs, oximetry, and capnography are best recorded automatically, to avoid an optimistic interpretation later. Drugs, doses, route of administration, and timing must also be noted. Injuries are recorded as they are identified in anatomical order. Ischaemic times and entrapment times are important.

> **Anaesthesia is a useful prehospital technique, but should be used only by clinicians with appropriate training**

HEMS record chart.

The figure of the cervical collar is published by permission of Mr James King Holmes, and those of the pulse oximeter and CO_2 analysers and the KED extrication device were taken by the Department of Medical Illustration, Salford Royal Hospitals NHS Trust.

21 TRANSPORTATION TO HOSPITAL

Carl L Gwinnutt, Alastair W Wilson, Peter Driscoll

Timing and type of transport are governed by the patient's injuries and response to resuscitation. After extraction, the patient may be stabilised at the accident site before transportation by road ambulance to hospital. Although speed is of the essence, the time taken to secure the airway, institute effective ventilation, control bleeding, gain intravenous access, and splint the spine and limbs, is time well spent. As a doctor can do many more interventions than a paramedic, and the task is to restore normal physiological variables where possible, it is important that protocols are not restrictive. Nevertheless, the doctor should aim at moving within 15 minutes. The "Platinum 10 minutes" used as a guide by the British Association of Immediate Care is a good target.

If it is impossible to stabilise the patient at the scene without complex intervention, the patient must be transported to the closest appropriate hospital by the fastest possible transport with continuous resuscitation. The most common cause of instability is uncontrollable haemorrhage. Remember that external cardiac compression does not work on an empty heart and survival after hypovolaemic arrest at the scene is a rarity.

Delays in the transport of patients to multidisciplinary units from non-specialist hospitals are usual, so it pays to take the patient to the right hospital directly from the accident site. This triage decision must be made in the light of local specialty availability, the mechanism of injury, and an assessment of anatomical injuries.

> **Before transportation check that**
>
> - The airway is clear and secure and the spine is secure
> - Breathing is normal and ventilation symmetrical
> - Two intravenous lines are running adequately
> - All monitors are functioning
> - Drugs and equipment are accessible

Packaging and stabilisation

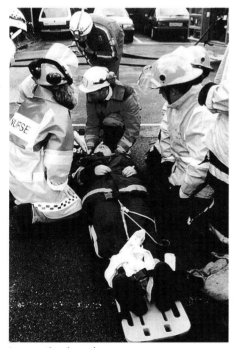

Long spine board.

Two principles underpin transportation; the first is to do no further harm and the second is "to anticipate a disaster with every transfer". All movement subjects the injured patient to energy changes which are inherently harmful. Movement of fractured limbs is painful and any movement of the head, neck, or thorax may result in dislocation of a precarious spine with further injury to the cord. Even the internal organs of a fully immobilised patient are subjected to inertial forces which exacerbate injury. Consequently, if an unrestrained patient in the back of a speeding ambulance moves about as it brakes, accelerates, or corners, further damage is inevitable. In addition, appreciable energy changes occur as stretchers are manhandled into vehicles, so from start to finish the journey should be as smooth as possible.

Managing the patient in the lateral position, though ideal in some respects, is inappropriate if a spinal injury has not been excluded. The whole spine must be protected. Most patients are transported supine, usually on a long spine board or a Vacumat™ mattress. This allows patients to be tipped or turned if they start to vomit. The risks of this can be reduced by inserting a nasogastric or orogastric tube but this is not a substitute for having suction at hand.

Pregnant patients should be transported in such a way as to displace the uterus to the left to prevent the supine hypotension syndrome (see chapter 17). Confused patients must be adequately restrained once cerebral hypoxia has been eliminated. If this proves impossible anaesthesia with paralysis may be indicated.

The airway is most effectively protected with a well secured cuffed tracheal tube. Consideration should be given to inserting one in an unconscious patient who is tolerating an oropharyngeal airway, or one with inhalation burns, particularly if faced with a long journey. Where

Transportation to hospital

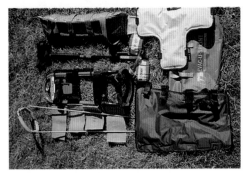

Variety of limb splints.

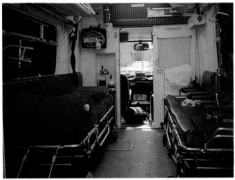

Interior of land ambulance.

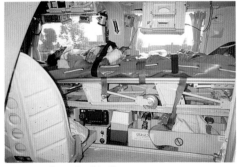

Interior of medical helicopter.

Equipment carried on medical helicopters

- Non-invasive blood pressure monitor
- Electrocardiograph and pulse rate monitor
- Invasive blood pressure monitors
- Temperature monitors
- Pulse oximeter and pulse rate monitor
- Capnograph
- Defibrillator
- Syringe drivers and infusion pumps
- Ventilators
- Suction

there is considerable likelihood of an unstable cervical spine, remember the possibility of nasal intubation and the surgical creation of an airway (see chapter 3).

A high inspired oxygen concentration may need to be maintained, and if you are using a portable mechanical ventilator remember that in many the same oxygen source is used to drive the machine as is supplying the patient. Consequently, small cylinders will empty quickly and a disconnect alarm as with the PAC is a useful safety measure.

Patients with a needle thoracocentesis in situ, or a simple pneumothorax or haemothorax, should have a large bore chest drain inserted and connected to a drainage system before transport.

The patient at risk of hypovolaemic shock requires two functioning large bore intravenous cannulas which must be secured. If they have been inserted in the antecubital fossa, an Armback splint keeps the arm straight. Central venous access at the scene of an accident is seldom indicated.

Limb splinting

The aim of splinting is to reduce blood loss, prevent soft tissue damage, and provide pain relief. A variety of non-compromising traction splints are available which allow inspection of the limb and palpation of pulses. Conforming vacuum splints that can be moulded around the patient's limbs are helpful. Whole body splinting can, to some extent, be achieved with the semirigid Evacumat splints.

Pneumatic Anti-Shock Garments (PASG), are useful for controlling continued haemorrhage from pelvic fractures (and intra-abdominal bleeding). They must not be used in patients with pulmonary oedema, ruptured diaphragm, or uncontrolled bleeding above the level of the abdomen. They are not a substitute for giving intravenous fluids.

Monitoring during transportation

The transport phase should no longer be regarded as a therapeutic vacuum. Paramedic ambulances and medical helicopters are designed to facilitate therapeutic manoeuvres on the move. This requires space, lighting, access to the patient, and availability of equipment.

Ideally the patient should be positioned with his or her head next to the attendant's seat and there must be room to gain access to the airway to allow tracheal intubation. It should be possible to identify and relieve a tension pneumothorax in a ventilated patient. Additional intravenous lines may be established and fractures splinted. If there is cardiac arrest cardiopulmonary resuscitation is difficult for a single operator, and is more effective when done by two attendants.

One of the most important tasks of the medical attendant during transportation is the continued monitoring and assessment of the patient. Heart rate, respiratory rate, systolic blood pressure, oximetry, and capnography may be continuously recorded and the level of consciousness must be assessed regularly.

Land ambulances

A compromise between speed and safety is required. The speed of an ambulance flashing a blue light is only marginally faster than its routine speed. Two tone sirens terrify patients, as well as the passing motorist. Consider the wisdom of the "go faster" approach.

Air ambulance

The designated medical helicopter is the most expensive part of the evacuation armamentarium and should be used with care. The crew should be trained to the highest possible level and must act as the extended arm of the hospital. As the helicopter can be used for long and short transportation in addition to secondary transport from primary hospitals to tertiary multidisciplinary centres, it requires full monitoring facilities.

Helicopters that are not specifically designed for medical transportation (police or military aircraft) may have only minimal medical equipment. The use of non-tested monitoring and defibrillation equipment can interfere with an aircraft's avionics, and radio transmissions can look like ventricular fibrillation (VF) on the monitor, with a possibly fatal outcome. Some are cramped, making management of the patient difficult.

Helicopter transport

Indications
- Need for specialist trauma centre care
- Long distances
- Obstruction to land transport by traffic
- Obscure or inaccessible accident sites
- Interhospital transfer of critically ill patients
- Transportation of medical staff or equipment to accident scene

Contraindications
- Weather
- Difficulty in landing because of obstruction or poor lighting
- Patient's injuries do not warrant care in specialised unit
- Patients who are violent or have psychiatric problems
- Incident is close to the most appropriate hospital for the patient's needs

Anticipating potential problems is even more important than during land transport and potential problems are best solved before lift off. Ensure that all the necessary equipment, and space to cope with emergencies, are available during flight.

Helicopters are noisy, which makes communication difficult and the use of a stethoscope impossible. Headphones should be placed on the patient's head to allow reassuring conversation. The patient must be kept warm and comfortable during the flight. If a long journey is expected an antiemetic may be given to prevent air sickness and the stomach should be kept empty by gastric aspiration.

Communication and handover

Essential information given en route to the receiving hospital

- The number of patients
- Age and sex of the patients
- Mechanism of injury
- Vital signs at the scene
- Initial findings on assessment
- Procedures at scene
- Response to treatment given
- Estimated time of arrival

Staff in the receiving hospital must be informed of the patient's impending arrival and condition by either the ambulance staff or the accompanying medical attendant. In the light of the information received, staff in the emergency department can prepare the resuscitation room and call the trauma team (see chapter 1).

On arrival, details about the accident, the patient's initial condition, treatment given, and response, must be communicated to the appropriate member of staff. It is particularly important that problems that have occurred during transportation should be communicated, along with improvements or deteriorations in vital signs since resuscitation. Prehospital care personnel must wait to ensure that the team leader has all the necessary information.

Transfer between hospitals

On leaving, collect all equipment.

After major injuries patients may have to be transferred to another hospital. Arrangements must be made between doctors initiating and receiving the transfer. A decision about the minimal level and specialty of accompanying personnel must be made at this time, because unstable, ventilated patients require high levels of medical and anaesthetic support. The patient must be fully stabilised.

Provision should be made for all requirements during transfer, including adequate amounts of intravenous fluid, blood, supplementary drugs, and kit for reintubation and replacement of lines. Humidification should be provided on long journeys to prevent secretions blocking the tube. The nasogastric or orogastric tube should be suctioned regularly and the urinary catheter monitored for output. Take the patient's records and the results of all investigations. If possible, take original copies of *x* ray films and computed tomography so that they do not have to be repeated. Where possible maintain communication with the receiving hospital.

On arrival, the patient should be handed over to the receiving doctor with a resume of the history, treatment, and results. Problems encountered en route and action taken are important. All documentation should be handed over and equipment retrieved before leaving. Nothing is more embarrassing than returning home with the patient's *x* ray films and without the Propac monitor.

Further reading

Reeve WG, Runcie CJ, Reidy J, Wallace PGM. Current practice in transferring critically ill patients among hospitals in the west of Scotland. *BMJ* 1990; **300**: 85–91.
Guidelines for the transfer of critically ill patients. *Crit Care Med* 1993; **21**: 931–7.
British Association for Immediate Care. *Prehospital emergency care.* Edinburgh: Royal College of Surgeons of Edinburgh, 1994.
Nancekievill DG. On site medical services at major incidents. *BMJ* 1992; **305**: 726–7.

22 MANAGEMENT OF SEVERE BURNS

Colin Robertson, Oliver Fenton

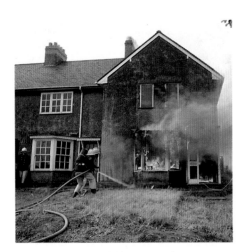

At the scene of a fire first aid procedures are often life saving. Medical staff should use the following instructions for preparing a victim for evacuation to a burns unit. Under the direction of the fire service and ensuring the safety of the rescuers the patient should be removed from the scene of injury to a place of safety and fresh air.

Flames and heat track upwards, so the patient should be kept supine and rolled or covered with a heavy blanket, coat, or rug to extinguish any residual flames. Take care not to get burnt yourself, especially if dealing with petrol burns or self immolation.

If the clothing is still smouldering or hot apply large amounts of cold water. Clothing saturated with boiling liquids or steam should be removed rapidly, but do not remove burnt clothing that is adherent to the skin. Cover burnt areas with clean (sterile if available) towels or sheets and ensure that the patient is kept warm. **Do not apply wet soaks or ice packs or use them during transit** as this will not provide any pain relief for patients with full thickness burns and can cause profound hypothermia, especially in children.

Evacuate the patient to the receiving hospital as quickly as possible. In patients with severe burns or those who have been exposed to smoke or fumes high flow oxygen through a facemask should be given during transit. Alert the receiving accident and emergency department by radio or telephone as to the number and ages of the patients and the severity of their burns, together with the estimated time of arrival.

Reception and resuscitation

Necessary information on incident

- Its nature (house fire, blast, release of steam or hot gas, etc)
- If possible, the nature of burning materials (furniture, polyurethane foam, polyvinyl chloride, etc)
- Was there any explosion?
- Was the patient in an enclosed space?
- For how long was the patient exposed to smoke or fire?
- The time elapsed from burn/injury/smoke inhalation to arrival in hospital.

The primary assessment, investigation, and treatment of a patient with severe burns should be a continuous and integrated process rather than a stepwise progression. While assessment is being performed a member of staff must obtain the necessary information about the incident from the ambulance crew and other emergency services. This should then be conveyed to the senior doctor in charge of the patient.

Management of the airway

Clinical features indicating smoke or thermal injury to respiratory tract

Altered consciousness

Direct burns to face or oropharynx

Hoarseness, stridor

Soot in nostrils or sputum

Expiratory rhonchi

Dysphagia

Drooling, dribbling, and saliva

Rapidly examine the patient for clinical evidence of smoke inhalation and thermal injury to the respiratory tract. In patients with one or more of the features described in the box respiratory obstruction from pharyngeal or laryngeal oedema may develop rapidly. Patients exposed to steam or hot vapours are at particular risk of damage to the upper airways. Stridor, difficulty in swallowing, and drooling of saliva are signs of epiglottic swelling. In such patients examination and early endotracheal intubation performed by an experienced doctor with anaesthetic training is essential. Mucosal swelling of the oropharynx and epiglottis can be extremely rapid, and delay can render tracheostomy necessary. In patients in whom complete respiratory obstruction has already occurred or intubation is unsuccessful, or both, immediate cricothyrotomy or "mini" tracheostomy is required, followed by formal tracheostomy. It should be emphasised, however, that in patients with severe burns the tracheostomy site is an important site of infection.

All patients suspected of having thermal or smoke injury to the respiratory tract should be given humidified high flow oxygen (an inspired oxygen concentration (FiO_2) of at least 40%–60%) through a facemask. If bronchospasm is present give the patient a β_2 agonist (such as salbutamol or terbutaline) with an oxygen powered nebuliser.

Frequent repeated clinical assessment of the airway and ventilation is mandatory in patients with all types of injuries caused by fire, together with further measurements of arterial blood gas tensions, carboxyhaemoglobin and, if the patient can comply, peak expiratory flow rates. Note that measurement of oxygen saturation by pulse oximetry may give erroneous readings in the presence of carboxyhaemoglobin.

Intravenous access

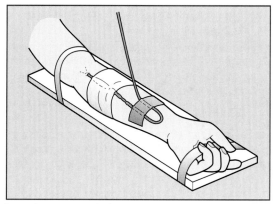

Intravenous cannulation.

Establishing adequate intravenous access must not be delayed. Insert and secure one or more large bore (needle gauge 14–16) intravenous cannulas. If possible use 10–15 cm cannulas to reduce the risk of dislodgement. The normal and easiest sites for percutaneous insertion of intravenous cannulas are the forearms and antecubital fossae. Narrow bore cannulas inserted into small veins on the back of the hands are of little practical value. Occasionally, alternative sites such as the external jugular and femoral veins or the long saphenous vein at the ankle must be used, although the saphenous vein is prone to early occlusion.

Intravenous cutdown in the cubital fossae or on the long saphenous vein in the groin may be required if percutaneous intravenous access cannot be performed. This approach can be made through burnt skin, but if this is the case do not attempt to suture the resulting gaping wound. If possible, before attaching the tubing of the intravenous drip take enough blood through the cannula for crossmatching and determining blood group, packed cell volume, and urea and electrolyte concentrations.

Intravenous fluid requirements

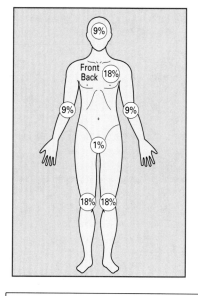

For rapid assessment the "rule of nine" is useful. Do not include areas of simple erythema in the estimate. The size of small burns can be judged roughly by considering the palmar surface of the patient's closed hand as about 1% of the total body surface area. Use your own hand to map out the burnt area, and then make allowances for the size of your hand compared with the patient's—for example, it would be three times the size of a 1 year old child's and twice the size of a 5 year old child's. The result can be cross checked by mapping the size of the unburnt area. In patients with very large burns it is simpler to measure the unburnt area and then subtract from 100.

Example

Weight of patient who has sustained a burn = 70 kg

Body surface area covered = 35%

Volume of colloid required in first four hours after injury $= \dfrac{35 \times 70}{2}$

$= 1225$ ml

Start treatment with intravenous fluids; the first 500 ml should be 0.9% saline. If colloid is then used—for example, 5% albumin, gelatin, or dextran solutions—the volume of fluid required for intravenous replacement treatment for the first four hours since injury should be judged roughly as the percentage of the body surface area of the burn multiplied by the body weight (kg) divided by two.

Patients with full thickness burns that cover >10% of the body surface area may require a transfusion of red blood cells in addition to fluid replacement. A blood transfusion is given in place of the colloid requirement for that period. In major burns the blood would have to be given during the resuscitation period, but in smaller burns it may be given at the end of resuscitation.

Management of severe burns

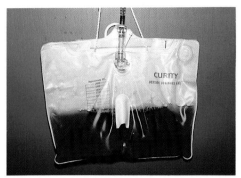

Urine from a patient with electrical burns indicates haemoglobinuria.

Insert a urinary catheter and start hourly measurements of urine volume. Note the colour and consistency of the initial urine in patients with severe flame or high voltage electrical burns. The urine may be a treacly black, indicating haemoglobinuria or myoglobinuria, or both. This is of prognostic importance for subsequent renal function.

In elderly patients, patients with cardiorespiratory disease, and patients who have delayed presentation consider inserting a central venous pressure line if you are experienced in the technique. This can play an important part in the subsequent restoration of volume in a patient with a severe burn. The risks of infection related to a central line are small in the early stages. With current methods of line management these risks are outweighed by the importance of the line for monitoring and access.

Analgesia and reassurance

> **Pain relief in patients with severe burns**
>
> *Entonox*—for conscious, cooperative patients, especially in the prehospital phase
>
> *Opioids*—give intravenously in small aliquots titrated to the patient's clinical response

The rate of intravenous fluid replacement should be tailored by the above guideline and the clinical response of the patient in terms of haemodynamic variables and urine output. The aim in adults is to achieve a urine output of 0.5–1.0 ml/kg/hour.

Severe burns cause both pain and distress. Analgesia and reassurance should be given as soon as possible. Treatment for pain in patients with severe burns must be tailored to the patient's individual requirements. Full thickness burns, if present, are pain free, but all patients will be frightened and distressed, and constant reassurance and communication are vital.

A mixture of 50% nitrous oxide and 50% oxygen (Entonox) given by an on demand system with a tight fitting facemask can provide simple and effective analgesia, particularly before arrival in hospital. Subsequently, if required, an opioid such as Cyclimorph (cyclizine and morphine) should be given intravenously in aliquots of 1 mg at a dose carefully titrated to the clinical response.

Reassessment

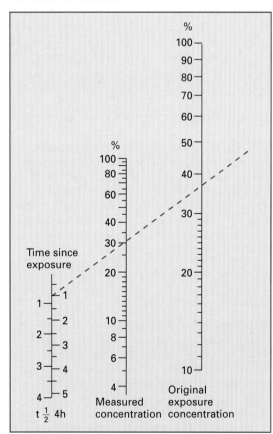

Nomogram for calculating carboxyhaemoglobin concentration at time of exposure.

Time since exposure is given in two scales to allow for effects of previous oxygen administration as half life of carboxyhaemoglobin (left scale assumes a half life of 3 h).

The airway

Confirm that the patient's airway is secure and that ventilation is adequate. Repeat the measurements of arterial blood gas tensions and the analysis of carboxyhaemoglobin concentrations, which give an approximate guide to the amount of smoke inhaled; concentrations at the time of exposure can be predicted by using the nomogram. For example, if the carboxyhaemoglobin concentration is 30% one hour after exposure the concentration at exposure would have been about 37%.

Clinical features of carbon monoxide poisoning correlate only moderately well with carboxyhaemoglobin concentrations but alteration of the conscious state should be regarded with suspicion. The so called "classic" feature of cherry red mucous membranes is a rarely seen, totally unreliable clinical sign.

Treatment with hyperbaric oxygen may be indicated in patients with carboxyhaemoglobinaemia particularly if they are or have been unconscious, have cardiac or neurological symptoms, or are pregnant. Early consultation with local hyperbaric specialists is recommended.

Other toxic gases, such as hydrogen cyanide, hydrogen sulphide, and hydrogen chloride, are often produced in fires. They may cause local irritation to both upper and lower airways as well as acting systemically as direct cellular poisons. Few laboratories can provide cyanide concentrations in an emergency, but a severe metabolic acidosis, high lactate concentration, and an increased anion gap suggest cyanide poisoning if there is an appropriate history of exposure. In these patients emergency resuscitation with assisted ventilation is required, and the use of cyanide antidotes (such as sodium thiosulphate with amyl nitrite (for enhanced distribution), and dicobalt edetate) should be considered.

Ensure that deep circumferential burns of the thorax are not causing restriction in chest expansion and hence ventilation (see below).

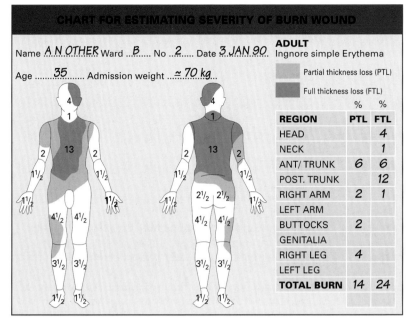

CHART FOR ESTIMATING SEVERITY OF BURN WOUND

Name *A N OTHER* Ward *B* No *2* Date *3 JAN 90*

Age *35* Admission weight *≃ 70 kg*

ADULT
Ignore simple Erythema

REGION	PTL %	FTL %
HEAD		4
NECK		1
ANT/ TRUNK	6	6
POST. TRUNK		12
RIGHT ARM	2	1
LEFT ARM		
BUTTOCKS	2	
GENITALIA		
RIGHT LEG	4	
LEFT LEG		
TOTAL BURN	**14**	**24**

Partial thickness loss (PTL)
Full thickness loss (FTL)

Lund and Browder chart.

Treatment with fluids

The rule of nine, which is used in the rapid assessment of the burn injury, can result in overestimation of the extent of the burn. More accurate assessment can be made with Lund and Browder charts and the rate of intravenous replacement adjusted accordingly.

Formulas for intravenous fluid requirements are, however, only rough guides and need modification according to the patient's clinical state. Regular checks and recording of pulse rate, blood pressure, central venous pressure (if indicated), urine output, packed cell volume, and peripheral perfusion and of the trends in their values can provide additional guidance for adjusting the rate of infusion.

Contrary to expectations, fluid replacement should not be limited in patients with burns and inhalation injury. Indeed, increased fluids are often needed to maintain the systemic circulation and optimise cardiac and renal function.

The burns

Pending the patient's transfer from the accident and emergency department to the ward or specialist burns unit the burnt area should be covered with a sterile, warm, non-adherent dressing. A layer of Clingfilm covered by a dry sheet and blanket is effective. Under no circumstances should a patient be transferred in wet sheets or towels as this can lead to hypothermia, with occasional fatal consequences.

Deep circumferential burns over the limbs, neck, and chest can produce a tourniquet like effect as the damaged skin is unable to expand as tissue oedema develops. If this occurs escharotomies (longitudinal incisions of the skin) are required to permit adequate circulation and ventilation. Circumferential neck burns may also make intubation difficult and so escharotomy is required. It is often necessary to do escharotomies before transfer. The affected part should be incised under sterile conditions on both sides just as a plaster of Paris cast is bivalved. Ensure that the entire length of the constriction is released. In the hand take the incisions right to the tips of affected digits.

If escharotomy of the chest is required vertical incisions along anterior and posterior axillary lines should be made. If sufficient chest expansion does not occur further incisions in the midline and midclavicular lines and transverse incisions may be required. Escharotomy does not require anaesthesia as the burns are full thickness burns. If it does cause pain then escharotomy is probably not indicated.

Failure to do an early escharotomy can lead to the loss of a limb; therefore if doubtful always err on the side of escharotomy. The incisions do not cause any additional scarring as the burns are full thickness. Substantial bleeding occurs from the wounds, and sterile absorbent dressings should be applied and, if necessary, blood replacement given. Ensure that the patient is adequately protected against tetanus.

Lethal burns

Although improvement in the management of burns in intensive care is resulting in a number of patients surviving burns of more than 90% of the total body surface area, it is still the case that few patients survive full thickness burns of more than 70% of the total body surface area. As a rough guide, if the patient's age added to the percentage of the body surface area of the burn exceeds 100 the chances of survival are less than 50%. Any decision not to treat a patient with a lethal burn aggressively must be taken by a consultant with experience in burns. If aggressive resuscitation is not to be instituted in a patient the other aspects of reassurance and analgesia are of even greater importance. Remember that even patients with 100% full thickness burns are usually conscious and sentient.

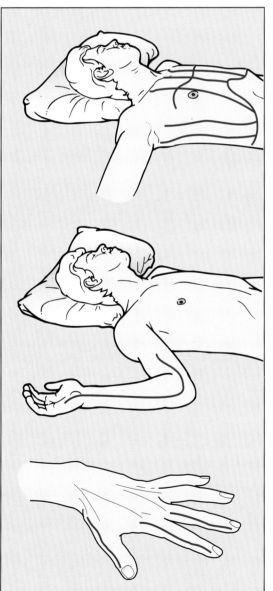

Escharotomy of the chest, arm, and fingers.

Management of severe burns

General aspects

Ask the patient and the relatives about pre-existing medical conditions, especially if these may be relevant to the therapeutic intervention being performed—for example, obstructive airways disease and ischaemic heart disease. Consider the possibility of underlying medical conditions that may have led to the burn injury—for example, epilepsy, a cerebrovascular episode, hypoglycaemia, drug or alcohol overdose.

In elderly patients, patients with known ischaemic heart disease, and all patients with a carboxyhaemoglobin concentration >15% obtain a 12 lead electrocardiogram and attach a cardiac monitor. Myocardial ischaemia or infarction and arrhythmias occur commonly and often do not have their usual clinical features.

Consider the possibility of non-accidental injury in children.

Do not give prophylaxis with antibiotics or steroids.

Depending on local policies discuss the patient's management with the burns or plastic surgical receiving team. If the patient is being transported within the hospital or to another referral hospital adequate intravenous fluids and analgesics should be transported along with him or her. All patients suspected of having inhaled smoke or requiring additional care of the airway must be escorted by an experienced anaesthetist with appropriate equipment.

Make clear, concise notes, which must accompany the patient and should include the size of the burn; the weight of the patient; the time when intravenous fluids were started; which drugs were given for pain relief and at what dose and time they were given; the urine and fluids chart; and details of special problems.

Chemical burns

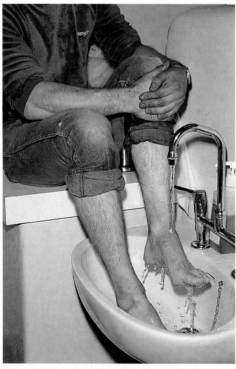

Chemical burn being copiously washed under a tap.

In an emergency all chemical burns can be treated with copious quantities of water and a bar of soap applied as soon as possible after the injury. Although there are specific treatments for certain chemicals (see below) these may be difficult to recall with accuracy in a confused environment and water and soap applied urgently in sufficient quantity for sufficient time will cover all eventualities.

Running water should be applied for at least 20 minutes, and should be lukewarm rather than cold if possible. The soap is not always necessary, but will overcome difficulties with organic chemicals (such as phenol) that may not be soluble in water.

In most factories that deal with dangerous chemicals buffer solutions are available and procedures exist for neutralising specific agents. In some cases, however, these injuries may be first seen in an accident and emergency department and some of those from more common substances will benefit from specific treatment.

Hydrofluoric acid

This is used in the glass industry and for cleaning pipes and is both toxic and painful. It can be neutralised by calcium gluconate gel or, in more severe cases, the calcium gluconate may be injected as a 10% solution under the skin to prevent further tissue damage and relieve the pain.

Phenol (carbolic acid)

This is an organic acid so is not readily soluble in water, but it can be removed rapidly with ethylene glycol (antifreeze). Like hydrofluoric acid phenol can not only cause local damage but is also a systemic poison, and as with many chemical burns the prognosis usually depends more on the systemic effects of absorption than on the surface area of the burn.

White phosphorus

This is used in the manufacture of explosives, and continues to burn when in contact with air. Particles may become embedded in the skin and have to be covered with water to prevent further combustion. A dilute solution of copper sulphate added to the water will make the phosphorus go black which makes it easier to identify and remove.

Electrical burns

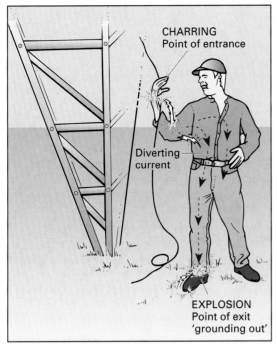

CHARRING
Point of entrance

Diverting
current

EXPLOSION
Point of exit
'grounding out'

Patient receiving a high voltage electrical injury, entering through the hand and grounding out through the foot.

A clear distinction should be made between flash and contact electrical burns. **Flash** electrical burns result in a high dry air temperature for a brief period of time which produces a superficial charring of the skin. This is almost always less severe than it looks and usually heals without the need for grafting unless there has been associated thermal injury from clothing that has caught fire. **Contact** electrical burns are the result of an electric current passing through the tissues and damaging the tissue in its passage. These burns are almost always worse than they look because much of the damage may be in the deeper tissues in spite of a relatively minor injury visible on the skin.

Contact electrical burns are usually divided into low voltage and high voltage, the dividing point being 1000 volts. In practice this means the difference between household and industrial currents, and the distinction may help in deciding how severe an injury is likely to be. Lethal injuries do, however, occur at household voltages. Voltage is the only variable that may be gleaned from the history as density of current, resistance, and time of exposure will not be known. Alternating current (mains) can provoke a tetanic contracture of the muscles which makes it difficult to release the contact. Direct current (lightning) tends to throw the injured person away. In an emergency **never** attempt to pull somebody off a current source unless you are **certain** that the current has been switched off or the person is pulled off with an insulated agent such as a dry wooden stake.

The damage caused by the passage of an electric current is caused by the heat generated by the current which is related to the density of the current, the resistance of the tissues through which the current passes, and the volume of tissue through which the current passes. Dry skin offers a high resistance and can therefore generate high temperatures with obvious tissue damage. If the current passes through a large contact area both in and out of the body, however, there may be no visible skin injury; this is seen when a large contact plate is used in unipolar diathermy. Therefore, though an electrical contact will produce entry and exit points, it is not like a bullet wound in that the visible damage at either site will be related to the contact surface area.

An electrical current will follow the path of least resistance and will travel in as direct a line as possible between the points of contact, of which there must be at least two (source and earth) to form a circuit. A current that passes from the palm to the dorsum of the same hand will not deviate to affect the myocardium or brain, but a current that passes from hand to hand or hand to foot will almost certainly affect the myocardium; this may produce arrhythmias that must be carefully monitored and treated if necessary. With high voltages arcing injuries may occur in which the current will jump from forearm to upper arm or upper arm to chest causing thermal skin injuries at each site.

A current that is forced to travel through tissues of low cross-sectional area or volume (for example, a finger) or through tissues of high resistance (for example, bone) will generate temperatures that can reach thousands of degrees Celsius and cause severe tissue damage even though the overlying skin looks normal.

Contact electrical burns should be treated with respect and usually the patient should be admitted to hospital for observation or treatment by appropriate staff. If there is any possibility of myocardial damage, and in all lightning injuries, patients should be monitored with an electrocardiogram because delayed arrhythmias may occur.

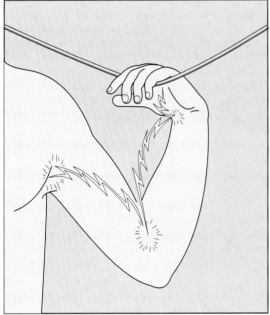

Arcing injury, between wrist, cubital fossa, and axilla.

The nomogram was reproduced with kind permission from the paper by C J Clark *et al.* (*Lancet* 1981;i:1332–5).

23 CHEMICAL INCIDENTS

Virginia Murray

Major chemical accidents cause problems for accident and emergency departments that are different from those recognised in other major incidents—for example, identification of the toxin, the risk of cross chemical contamination of staff and difficulties in patient management such as the need for specific antidotes. Particular attention should therefore be given to preparation and planning.

What is a chemical incident?

A chemical incident is the accidental or intentional release, or impending release, of a hazardous material. This chapter is concerned only with the response by accident and emergency departments to acute chemical incidents in which:

- the agent involved is present in large quantities or is potentially of high toxicity, or
- a large number of people are exposed or at risk of being exposed, or
- a large geographical area is at risk.

What are the local chemical hazards?

Accident and emergency departments may find it useful to strengthen their links with local emergency services such as the fire brigade and local and county authorities, including the emergency planning officers. The departments may need to develop new links with local Health and Safety Executive officers and local companies to identify factories or sites where hazardous substances may be manufactured, used, stored, transported, or disposed. In England, accident and emergency departments are required to cooperate with the new *Health Service Guidelines HSG(93)38* dated 20 August 1993 which delegate responsibility for coordinating the health aspects and response to chemical incidents to the local district health authority through a designated officer.

Many of these agencies will have information on methods of assessment, control, and mitigation in the event of accidents, much of which concludes with "seek medical advice." Few of them have experience in acute medical toxicology, and as a result they rely on advice from accident and emergency departments, who in turn rely on poisons centres such as the National Poisons Unit, London.

How can poisons centres help?

Poisons centres are essential resources for the provision of information and advice related to the diagnosis and management of cases of poisoning and for the medical aspects of management of chemical accidents. Their telephone numbers should be readily available in the accident and emergency department.

Under certain circumstances poisons centres may notify and collaborate with other agencies concerned in investigation and epidemiological follow up and may be able to provide on site toxicological advice and support. Analytical toxicology services available from the National Poisons Unit, London, cover advice on appropriate collection and testing of samples and interpretation of the results.

Health effects from chemical incidents

Initial symptoms usually relate to, but are not confined to, the route of exposure—inhalation will cause respiratory effects, and skin and systemic effects may occur where the substance is absorbed.

Examples of recent chemical accidents

Fires

Plastics recycling plant	Thetford, Norfolk, 1991
Chemical plant	Ellesmere Port, Cheshire, 1994

Explosions

Chemical plant	Castleford, Yorkshire, 1992

Chemical releases

Chemical plant	Portished, Avon, 1990
Oil tanker at sea	*Braer*, Shetlands, 1993

Chemical spills

Causing water pollution	River Dee, 1984
Causing water pollution	River Severn, 1994
Direct contamination of water supply	Lowermoor, North Cornwall, 1988

Services provided by poisons centres

The principal functions of the National Poisons Unit, London, in the event of a chemical incident are:

- To respond to requests for information and advice to medical professionals managing cases
- To assess, as rapidly as possible, the nature of the chemical hazard, to assist in determining toxic risk, and to disseminate relevant toxicological information
- To provide advice on issues such as decontamination, treatment, analytical toxicology, case registration and follow up.

Most effects will appear within a few hours of exposure but some may be delayed. In particular, respiratory symptoms can be delayed for up to 60 hours after inhalation. Because effects may be delayed, it is important to identify and document all those who were exposed, or were suspected of having been exposed as early as possible.

Susceptible groups that are particularly at risk from a toxic exposure are the young, the old, pregnant women and their fetuses, and those who have chronic illnesses. The route of exposure is an important factor in predicting which illnesses will result in increased susceptibility—for example, patients with emphysema are particularly sensitive to respirable gases.

Multiple hazards such as fire may present a complicated picture with both trauma and toxic effects.

What accident and emergency facilities are required?

The accident and emergency department consultants, in consultation with the district health authority and the local ambulance service should decide what equipment and facilities are needed by the health service to manage patients who have been (actually or potentially) exposed to hazardous chemical(s) (HSG (93)38). Facilities for resuscitation, decontamination, investigation, treatment as well as short and long term follow up of those exposed should be identified. However, the facilities for decontamination are often inadequate. Other equipment should include suitable protective clothing. In addition, adequate training and rehearsals in the use of equipment and facilities are essential.

Actions

So that early toxic hazard assessment may be undertaken, the accident and emergency department must obtain as much information as possible about

- Chemical(s) involved
- Type of incident
- Route(s) of exposure
- Type(s) of initial clinical effects.

It is important to identify and document everybody who has been exposed to chemicals because some who are initially symptom free may develop symptoms or become concerned about the effects of exposure at a later date. Consequently, chemical accident triage requires a new category in addition to the usual triage categories.

Reports received at the National Poisons Unit indicate that few accident and emergency departments have sent medical teams to chemical incidents over the last four years. It is likely that the need for a mobile medical team will arise only where patients who have been exposed to chemicals are also injured. If undertaking on site support, the following should be considered:

At the site – protection of the mobile medical team is essential, though there is no single set of protective clothing suitable for protection against every hazardous chemical. Medical teams should follow the layout pioneered in Canada.

The emergency services control centres should advise the mobile medical team when it is safe to provide medical aid or triage and should stay in communication. Preferably only decontaminated casualties should be attended. (Decontamination facilities are provided only for fire brigade staff but may be used for other casualties at the fire brigade's discretion. These are usually suitable only for upright patients, however, and provide only cold water decontamination.) The management of physical injuries follows the routine already described, but for the benefit of the casualty and emergency responders, all contaminated clothing should be removed, bagged and sealed in double clear plastic bags, preferably at the incident site. In addition to other medical equipment, therefore, consider taking surgical gowns or other clothing for casualties.

Chemical contamination of skin and eyes may require prolonged irrigation or even immersion of the affected part: **the solution to pollution is dilution.**

Susceptible groups

- any person directly contaminated by a chemical or as a result of a chemical incident
- at-risk groups—young, old, chronically ill, pregnant women
- first responders, eg fire, police, ambulance and medical personnel
- environmental and other clean-up workers

Triage categories

RED   :Life threatening
YELLOW   :Urgent but can wait
GREEN   :Can delay treatment
WHITE   :Dead

??? any case reporting chemical contamination but not symptomatic on initial examination

---

"Clean"/support zone

Emergency Services Control Centres (and Mobile Medical Team)

Contamination control line

Contamination reduction zone

Personal decontamination station

Hot line

"Dirty"/exclusion zone

Emergency Service Personnel wearing personal protective equipment only

WIND DIRECTION

"Clean" and "dirty" zone control lines. Layout pioneered in Canada.

Chemical incidents

Telephone numbers of poisons centres

National Poisons Unit,
London	0171 635 9191
Belfast	01232 240503
Birmingham	0121 5543801
Cardiff	01222 709901
Dublin	0103 531 379966
Edinburgh	0131 2292477
Leeds	0113 2430715
Newcastle	0191 2325131

At the accident and emergency department – the above principles also apply to casualties arriving at hospital. Early notification of an incident and of any casualties allows final preparation of hospital decontamination facilities and protective clothing by senior staff to minimise any contamination hazard inside the hospital. Preparation for triage assessment of chemical exposure and toxic risk assessment will probably require poisons centre support. In addition, the medical staff may find it helpful to seek advice from other experts on and off the incident site. A list of such contacts should be held ready for use.

Arrangements should be made as early as possible to obtain antidotes if appropriate and to provide facilities for supportive care.

Collection of blood, urine, vomit, and other relevant biological samples is valuable for confirming exposure and dose received and should be carried out as soon as possible after an incident in consultation with the poisons centre.

When discharging people who have attended the accident and emergency department, it is important not to return any patient to a previously contaminated environment without checking that it is safe to do so.

Conclusion

Though the management of injuries sustained in a chemical incident remains the same as for injuries from any other cause, special preparations must be taken by both the mobile medical teams and the receiving accident and emergency department. These should be taken in conjunction with the designated officer of the district health authority and the emergency services. Remember that the poisons centres can provide invaluable advice.

24 BLAST AND GUNSHOT INJURIES

Tim Hodgetts, Ian Haywood, Jim Ryan, David Skinner

Injuries from explosions and bullets are now common throughout the world. Here we discuss the mechanisms of injury, the management of the scene of a bomb or a shooting, and the treatment of individual casualties.

Explosions

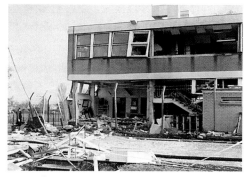

Bombing of Musgrave Park Hospital, November 1991.

Police role at the scene of an unexploded bomb

Confirm that there is a suspect device
Clear the area of people
Cordon to protect the scene
Control the incident

Remember the four Cs

Mechanisms of injury following a bomb

- Blast wave
- Blast wind
- Fragmentation (missiles)
- Flash burns
- Crush
- Psychological

A ruptured ear drum indicates exposure to an appreciable blast load:

- Is the patient deaf?
- Is the patient bleeding from the ears?

An explosion may be the result of a domestic accident (for example, household gas), or an industrial accident (for example, mining), but the principal cause outside a war zone is a terrorist bomb. Multiple casualties can be expected ranging from a handful to several hundred.

At the scene of an unexploded bomb the police will take charge. If doctors and nurses are deployed before the bomb explodes and can see the device they are clearly standing in the wrong place. Secondary devices are common after one explosion, and the scene should not be approached until it is declared safe by the police. Remember to check for a secondary device if people are to be moved from one area to another. Radio silence should be maintained initially to avoid triggering a radio-controlled bomb.

A bomb has six distinct mechanisms of injury:

- the blast wave
- the blast wind
- fragmentation
- flash burns
- crush
- psychological.

Blast wave

The blast wave is a front of overpressure formed by the compression of air at the interface of the rapidly expanding sphere of hot gases. The size of the overpressure falls off rapidly, and in proportion to the inverse of the distance cubed. With conventional "high" explosives such as trinitrotoluene (TNT) or Semtex (a "low" explosive is petrol or gunpowder which must be highly contained before they will explode) the blast wave will last only a few milliseconds. Injury is produced mainly by a combination of initial body compression (causing contusion of underlying solid organs), followed by then disruption of tissues at air/tissue interfaces (particularly in the lungs). Shearing forces then occur at tissue interfaces of different density (causing subserous and submucosal haemorrhage, particularly in the abdomen), and implosion of gas filled organs (causing acute perforation of intestine or tympanic membrane). The size of the overpressure can be multiplied several times over when the incident pressure is reflected by solid objects (such as ceiling or walls); the pressure wave will also be attenuated by water.

If air enters the pulmonary circulation as a result of disruption of the alveolar membrane, fatal coronary artery or cerebral artery air emboli may occur, possibly without external evidence of injury. Rupture of the eardrum is a useful clinical indicator that the patient has been exposed to an appreciable blast load, but the converse is not true if the drum is intact because the angle of the blast wave against the ear drum is thought to be critical.

Blast and gunshot injuries

The blast wave can produce two distinct patterns of lung injury. The common feature is intra-alveolar haemorrhage. There may be associated pneumothoraces and non fatal air emboli that may cause central nervous system signs (and may be seen in the retinal vessels). Although pulmonary injury is important, this "blast lung" is rare in those who survive to reach hospital (less than 1%).

By contrast, ischaemia of the bowel from subserous and submucosal haemorrhage can result in delayed perforation up to five days later which is usually heralded by abdominal pain and tenderness. Laparotomy should be reserved for those with clear signs of perforation (such as localised peritonitis or free air in the abdominal *x* ray film) because of the anaesthetic risk from the inevitable associated pulmonary injury.

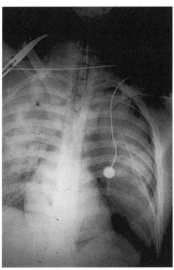

Radiograph of blast lung.

Blast winds

Blast winds are the rapidly moving displaced columns of air that follow the blast wave. They can be powerful enough to disintegrate and dismember anyone close to the point of the explosion. People who are further away or partly protected may sustain traumatic amputation of a limb; this sort of amputation, unlike a guillotine amputation, is usually unsuitable for reimplantation.

The wind may also throw people against solid objects, resulting in impact fractures or deceleration injuries. Debris of stone, glass, or broken street furniture carried in the wind will produce fragmentation missile injuries.

Fragmentation missiles

Most injuries after an explosion will be caused by fragmentation. They are caused by momentum (resulting in fractures and contusions), laceration, and penetration with high or low energy transfer (see below).

Flash burns

Such burns are usually superficial and of exposed skin. The possibility of smoke inhalation with upper airway involvement should always be considered.

Crush injuries

An explosion indoors may collapse the building on to the people inside, resulting in crush injuries.

Psychological injuries

Psychological injuries are the main objective of the terrorist. There will be short term panic and fear, and long term there will be post-traumatic stress disorder. Many more will have psychological scars than will sustain physical injuries, and symptoms of stress should also be watched for in carers both at the scene and at the hospital.

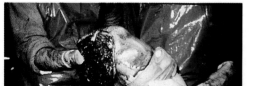

Traumatic amputation.

Penetrating missiles

Missile and bullet injuries

Important points:

- If chest penetration is possible, suspect and exclude tension pneumothorax
- Could the missile have injured the abdomen? If so, the prognosis is compromised and surgical exploration is usually essential. Administer broad spectrum antibiotics and tetanus prophylaxis early
- Wounds may be multiple, and patients may not be aware of all their injuries. Perform a thorough examination
- Suspect that minor wounds may contain foreign bodies. Perform radiography

Missiles include the primary and secondary fragments that follow an explosion, and bullets. Missile injuries from a bomb are often multiple, but the mechanism of injury and the management is the same whatever the cause.

The degree of injury that a missile produces depends on how much energy it imparts in the tissues. This in turn depends on how much energy the missile had to start with and how much it is retarded by the tissues. Because kinetic energy is the product of half the mass multiplied by the square of the velocity, a small missile travelling at high speed will maximise available energy. The density of the tissue and the type and stability of the missile will regulate the degree of retardation.

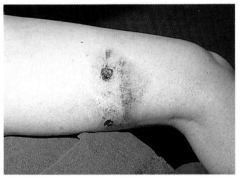

Simple gunshot wound.

Low energy transfer injuries

Missiles have traditionally been divided into "low velocity" and "high velocity," the arbitrary division being the speed of sound. More important, however, is the distinction between whether there has been high or low energy transfer to the wound. This is possible with either missile, but can be difficult to assess clinically even with a clear history. Nevertheless, low velocity missiles (such as from a handgun or large irregular fragments from an explosion) tend to produce injury only along the wound track by crushing and laceration (producing a "permanent cavity") with little damage away from the track. Death is likely only if a vital organ is damaged. Large irregular fragments are more readily retarded, and consequently will give up more energy.

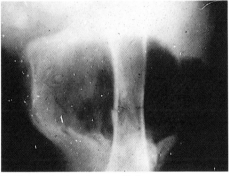

Radiograph showing cavitation.

High energy transfer injuries

High energy transfer missiles such as military rifle bullets also produce a permanent cavity, but the devastating injury seen in high energy transfer wounds can be a result of the temporary cavity which develops when the tissues continue to move away from the wound track after the missile has passed through. This produces a large cavity for a few milliseconds which then collapses and sucks in contaminated debris from the wound surface. Solid, semisolid, and abdominal hollow viscera can be disrupted; microscopically there are large areas of heterogeneous tissue damage, vascular instability, and some reversible ischaemia. If bone is struck there is nearly always high energy transfer and pieces of bone or broken missile can act as secondary missiles.

Management of injuries

In the resuscitation room

- Ensure safety. Check the patient for weapons
- Treatment priorities are airway, breathing, and circulation first
- Bag, seal, and label all of the patient's clothing and personal belongings. Secure these until handed to the police (to ensure continuity of evidence)
- Label any missile fragments found and hand them directly to the police
- If the patient is stable make notes of the position and size of all wounds (and retain a personal copy)

Safety is paramount at the scene of a bomb or shooting incident. In the emergency department always consider that the person who has been shot may also be carrying a gun: a hypoxic and confused patient with a gun is clearly a danger.

Resuscitation

Resuscitation of the injured follows the standard protocol of airway, breathing, and circulation. Ventilatory support may be needed for patients with blast lung, but this must be balanced against the theoretical increased short term risk of producing an air embolism. This can occur with intermittent positive pressure ventilation but is more likely with positive end expiratory pressure. Rapid transfer to the operating theatre for control of haemorrhage may be important with penetrating injuries.

Blast and gunshot injuries

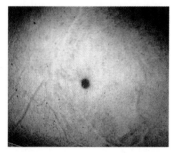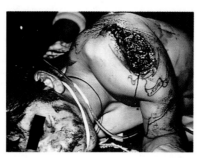

Shoulder wound caused by bomb fragment. Energy deposit damage and contamination (right) was found on exploration of what seemed to be a simple wound (left).

Contamination

All missile wounds are contaminated. With high energy transfer wounds, clothing can be disrupted into minute fragments and spread widely along tissue planes up to 20–30 cm distant from the wound track. These wounds are particularly susceptible to anaerobic infection with clostridia (tetanus and gas gangrene). With low energy wounds the plug of clothing is often closely associated with the missile.

High energy transfer wounds require aggressive surgery to remove dead tissue and foreign material and to ensure that no tension develops in the wound; this typically involves wide excision and fasciotomy.

Wounds are left open for delayed primary closure.

Immunity to tetanus must be ensured with immunoglobulin, or toxoid, or both. Antibiotics may help in preventing infection if given early, but there is no substitute for adequate surgery.

Conclusion

Management of blast injuries

- *Suspect*
If exposed to appreciable blast, even if no injury is apparent, observe the patient for 48 hours

- *Examine*
Initially follow standard ABC examination protocols, but also look for these specific injuries associated with exposure to a blast:

Chest	Examine for signs of respiratory failure and pneumothorax
	Do a chest x ray (Is there evidence of a pneumothorax? free gas under the diaphragm? signs of developing adult respiratory distress syndrome?)
Abdomen	Is there evidence of local peritonitis?
Central nervous system	Look for abnormal neurological signs (secondary to air emboli)
Funduscopy	Look for air emboli
Ears	Are the tympanic membranes perforated?
Olfactory function	The blast wave can produce anosmia through direct damage of the olfactory nerve endings. This has medicolegal consequences

- *Treat*
Confine the patient to a chair or bed to prevent exertion
Give high flow oxygen through a tight-fitting mask with reservoir
Maintain ventilation if there is respiratory failure, but balance this against the risk of embolism
If intermittent positive pressure ventilation is needed, consider prophylactic chest drains
Treat other injuries (amputation, missiles, burns) as necessary
Do laparotomy in cases of definite perforation

Gunshot and blast injuries are common worldwide, and an understanding of the mechanisms of injury is important in predicting clinical problems. Priorities in management are safety, airway, breathing, and circulation, before considering injuries specific to bombs or bullets.

25 TRAUMA IN HOSTILE ENVIRONMENTS

C J Cahill, Vanessa Lloyd-Davies

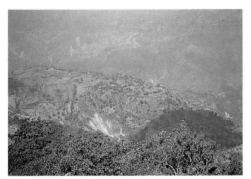

Foothills in eastern Nepal.

ABCDE of resuscitation

Airway and cervical spine
Breathing
Circulation and control of haemorrhage
Dysfunction of the central nervous system
Exposure

Most trauma in the United Kingdom is managed in a controlled environment, be it an accident and emergency department or an organised prehospital care system. The trauma team leader, in most circumstances, will be able to take control in the knowledge that he or she possesses appropriate equipment and expertise within the team, and that he or she can ensure rapid evacuation to a definitive care centre. In a hostile environment, however, this is not always the case.

In a war zone, the aftermath of an earthquake, or in a remote area, limited equipment, inclement working conditions, and uncertain evacuation will be coupled with the inherent dangers of the particular locality.

The conditions will undoubtedly affect how patients present, so a knowledge of the history of injury and the environment is even more important and will modify the management plan. It may be necessary to improvise according to the equipment available.

It must be emphasised that the priorities for patient assessment, triage and treatment remain the same: Airway, Breathing, Circulation, Disability, and Environment. Here, however, E also encompasses Evacuation. Full exposure may be impractical and dangerous and evacuation may have to take place before the secondary survey.

In this chapter we highlight some particular problems and give guidelines to assist in meeting the challenges they present.

General guidelines for hostile environments

The hostile environment:

- Will modify patient presentation
- Will affect your management
- Will necessitate improvisation
- But does not alter the priorities
    "ABCDE"

You may find yourself in a hostile environment unexpectedly, but if you are able to preplan then the following ABCs may assist in preparing you and your team.

A—Anticipation
Planning is the key. A thorough knowledge of the area and the conditions are essential; ideally use local knowledge, ensure you have up to date and accurate maps, and think of all the likely and unlikely eventualities. The "unexpected" will happen. Ask yourself if you really need to go into the area of risk. For example, tourists and "go it alone saviours" are not usually welcomed in disaster zones and risk becoming casualties themselves.

B—Backup
Ask yourself who is going to get you out if it all goes wrong and make sure that your backup team know where you are going to be and when you should be back. Do you have the appropriate clearances or approval and have you linked with other agencies involved in the same area and activities? Their expertise and experience might be essential to your success.

C—Communication
Poor communications often contribute to failure and disaster. Careful planning, appropriate equipment, and training must be considered. More than one method is desirable to minimise risks. The press, if present, can make useful allies but their priorities are different.

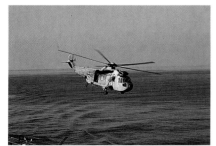

Helicopter rescue at sea.

Trauma in hostile environments

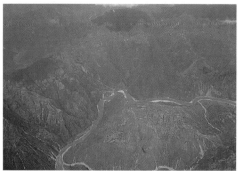

Mountainous territory, Nepal.

D—Danger

It is essential to assess the known risks and balance these against the benefits that you and your party can gain or offer. Appropriate safety equipment is essential as is training and knowledge. The aim is to avoid becoming a casualty yourself and to be self sufficient so that you do not become a burden to others.

E—Equipment

Keep it simple: the less technical it is the more likely it is to work. Plan the packing so you can get to an item when you need it and spread your resources evenly around your team to minimise the effect of loss of part of your kit. Stores should be broken down to reduce packing materials to a minimum and quantities should reflect your expected length of stay plus a reserve for emergencies. Remember, at all times, you have to be able to carry your stores.

Airway with cervical spine control

Airway

- Open
- Maintain
- Secure
- Cervical spine immobilisation as appropriate
- Nasopharangeal airway
- Cricothyroidotomy

Control of the airway is the first priority with cervical spine control, if appropriate. The aim is to open and maintain the airway and if necessary secure a definitive airway. Frequent reassessment is vital before and during evacuation. The history and mechanism of injury are important. If you suspect spinal injury then immobilise the spine, but needless immobilisation makes handling casualties more difficult and could endanger your patient. Improvisation is essential and relatively easy—for example, neck collar templates drawn on roll mats before departure, or sandbags made from socks filled with earth.

The following technical aspects should be considered. A nasopharyngeal airway may be better tolerated than an oropharyngeal one, and therefore require less supervision. Cricothyroidotomy may be more appropriate than intubation "in the field," as oral or nasal intubation is possible only if the patient is deeply unconscious. Sedation or paralysis, or both, may be difficult, and attempted nasal or oral intubation will raise intracranial pressure if the patient is conscious. The technique of cricothyroidotomy is simple and requires little equipment, but does require appropriately sized tubes (size 5/6).

Breathing

Breathing

- Thorough assessment
- Identify life threatening conditions
- Place and secure appropriate drains
- Conserve oxygen supplies
- Avoid under and over ventilation
- Reassess frequently

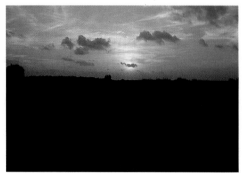

Sunrise in the desert.

Once you have established a patent airway, careful and thorough assessment of neck and chest, including the back, is required to ensure that the patient is breathing adequately. Look, feel, percuss, and listen, although this can be difficult in noisy environments. The aim is to identify and immediately treat life threatening conditions as well as to recognise potentially life threatening conditions so that you can minimise their effect until definitive investigation and treatment can be undertaken. Most life threatening chest injuries can be managed with an appropriately placed needle or tube. It is essential, therefore, to be able to do a needle thoracocentesis and to be able to insert a chest drain safely.

Remember to secure all tubes with sutures and tape. If a tube can fall out, it will fall out. Underwater seal drainage is not practical and flutter valves (Heimlick valves, Portex Emergency drainage bags) should be used. Be alert to the possibility that these devices may block with clotted blood.

Oxygenation is essential, but oxygen may be either limited or unavailable, as portable cylinders are heavy and last for a short time at high flows. Patient selection and conservation of valuable stocks is crucial. Give oxygen only when it is absolutely necessary. Consider the use of oxygen concentrators, if available, to conserve bottled gas supplies.

Manual or mechanical ventilation may be necessary but should be avoided if possible as without adequate monitoring there is a risk of hypercarbia or hypocarbia. If possible spontaneous respiration is preferable. Frequent reassessment and careful clinical monitoring are vital.

Circulation with control of haemorrhage

Circulation

- Assess carefully
- Limit haemorrhage
- Conserve intravenous fluids
- Consider hypotensive resuscitation
- Monitor response
- Remember preinjury losses

When are intravenous fluids required?

Class I haemorrhage
  <15% Oral (or rectal) fluids may be enough. Every effort must be made to control blood loss.

Class II haemorrhage
  15%–30% Oral (or rectal) fluids should be given, and careful monitoring is required. Intravenous access is essential and fluids may be required.
  Every effort must be made to control blood loss.

Class III haemorrhage
  30%–40% Intravenous fluids essential but with every effort to control blood loss. Improved level of consciousness, a palpable pulse, and urine output are your indicators of success.

Class IV haemorrhage
  >40% The casualty is in trouble and unless immediate evacuation and surgery are available. Your fluids may be better conserved for others.

In hostile environments a casualty is likely to have been exerting himself, or to have been exposed to extreme conditions before injury, and almost certainly he will already be depleted of fluid. A rapid overall assessment must be made taking account of this and the mechanism of injury, to estimate fluid requirements. Only minimal monitoring may be available, but clues can be obtained from simple observation, examination, and frequent reassessment—for example, a palpable radial pulse indicates a systolic blood pressure of greater than 80 mm Hg.

Supplies of intravenous fluids will almost certainly be at a premium and therefore conservation of those fluids must be an important consideration. Immediate operation to "turn off the tap" may not be an option. Thorough control of external haemorrhage is essential to avoid pouring in fluids only to have them lost from a bleeding wound, and "hypotensive" resuscitation should be considered. This aims to maintain perfusion of vital organs and hence oxygenation without increasing blood pressure to a point where further haemorrhage may result from loss of clot haemostasis.

Two large bore, short, peripheral cannulas should be placed if possible, by cutdown if necessary, and secured for later use if and when more fluids become available. Repeated percutaneous attempts at venous access merely wastes limited materials as well as time. Venous cutdown is a vital skill and with practise venous access can be achieved rapidly and reliably. Having obtained access securing the line is essential to prevent later problems: **if it can fall out it will**.

Colloid or crystalloid?

Classic advanced trauma life support teaching was formulated for the hospital environment where operating facilities and blood supplies are available. Blood is obviously the best fluid to replace blood lost but stored blood is unlikely to be available. Grouping your team before departure should be considered to provide a source of blood for transfusion but this requires that the equipment to bleed them should be carried too.

We suggest that a mixture of crystalloid and colloid be carried to provide a variety of responses to blood and fluid loss. Colloid takes up less space, stays in the circulation longer, and is required in lower volumes, but it is not appropriate for replacing simple fluid and electrolyte losses and may precipitate at low temperatures (<4°). Oral or rectal fluid, or both, can supplement intravenous fluids to cover basic requirements. Every fluid loss should be monitored and recorded if possible, to help to estimate requirements.

Disability

Disability

- Assess level of consciousness
- AVPU/GCS
- Reassess and record frequently
- Rapidly increasing intracranial pressure requires immediate evacuation

Neurological state must be assessed, monitored, and frequently reassessed to ensure optimum resuscitation and to diagnose and treat neurological injury. If there is neurological injury then the aim must be to prevent secondary injury resulting from less than adequate care. Major head injury in isolated and hostile environments carries an appalling prognosis as life saving surgical intervention is unlikely to be an option. Unless immediate evacuation is available, signs of rapidly increasing intracranial pressure presage death and it is likely that there is little that can be done. Diuretic treatment with mannitol will only delay the inevitable unless help is close at hand. Amateur neurosurgery is not to be recommended.

Good management of the ABCs with simple measures such as head up positioning are the mainstay of controlling intracranial pressure and preventing secondary brain injury.

Environment and evacuation

Environment

- Preplanning
- Good communications
- Appropriate transport
- Appropriate personnel
- Appropriate receiving facility
- Stabilise the patient
- Secure all lines and tubes

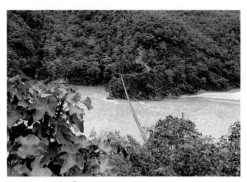

Tropical rain forest.

Each particular hostile environment presents its own problems and no list can be exhaustive; nevertheless, the following indicates the problems that can be encountered which make trauma care a serious challenge.

- *Desert*—Dry, with extremes of temperature (hot and cold).
    Problems: dehydration, lack of water supply, heat, cold, dust.
- *Disasters*—War, earthquake, famine, or flood.
    Problems: self preservation, food, clean water, easy to become a drain on others' resources.
- *Jungle*—Wet, hot.
    Problems: dehydration, clean water and food supply, endemic diseases.
- *Altitude*—Dry, wet, cold, and hypoxia.
    Problems: dehydration, exhaustion, altitude sickness, freezing cold injury.
- *Sea*—Wet, cold.
    Problems: dehydration, hypothermia, motion sickness, non-freezing cold injury.

Evacuation requires careful preplanning and preparation. After the catastrophe has occurred is the wrong time to start organising your way out. The key elements required to meet the challenge of trauma care in a hostile environment are a sound understanding of the principles of trauma care, anticipation, and above all flexibility.

We thank Professor J Ryan for allowing us to use the pictures of Nepal and the tropical rain forest.

26 MAJOR INCIDENTS

Tim Hodgetts, Stephen Miles

Date	Type	Incident	Casualties	
			Dead	Injured
6 July 1988	Industry	Piper Alpha	164	25
8 January 1989	Air	Kegworth (M1)	47	79
6 March 1987	Sea	Herald of Free Enterprise	137	402
12 December 1988	Rail	Clapham Junction	34	115
9 September 1987	Road	M4 crash	4	74
15 April 1989	Stadium	Hillsborough	95	200
20 March 1993	Terrorist bomb	Warrington	2	55

An incident is described as "major" when the number, severity, or type of live casualties, or the location of the incident, require extraordinary arrangements to be made by the NHS. Natural incidents (floods, hurricanes, tidal waves) still account for most of the deaths worldwide, but man made incidents (those resulting from technological or other human interaction) are more common. The potential for a man made incident exists whenever a large number of people gather together.

Preparation

The preparation for a major incident involves planning, training, and acquisition of equipment. Every hospital that may receive casualties must have a major incident plan which will detail the organisation and actions of staff both in hospital and at the scene. When making a major incident plan reference to the NHS Management Executive's *Emergency planning in the NHS* will be useful.[1]

The doctor in charge at the scene is the medical incident officer; doctors and nurses sent to treat patients at the scene under his direction are termed mobile medical teams. Doctors who may take on the role of medical incident officer at the scene must be given supplementary training in command and communications as well as gaining experience in prehospital care, in addition to training for their individual responsibilities. Any doctor at the scene is **not** necessarily better than no doctor at all. The Prehospital Emergency Care Certificate and the Diploma in Immediate Medical Care provide standards for training, but doctors should also take a specific course in the medical management of a major incident. Doctors and nurses who are members of the mobile medical team should also be trained in prehospital care and should understand their roles and the organisation of the scene.

Suggested staff training requirements

Medical Incident Officer
- Diploma in Immediate Medical Care (Royal College of Surgeons of Edinburgh) or Prehospital Emergency Care Certificate

and

- Major Incident Medical Management and Support (MIMMS) course (3 days) [*other major incident training courses available*]

and

- advanced life support instruction (Advanced Trauma Life Support/Prehospital Trauma Life Support)

Member of mobile medical team
- Prehospital Emergency Care course

and

- Major Incident Medical Management and Support (MIMMS) course (first 2 days only)

and

- advanced life support instruction (ATLS/PHTLS)

Major incident definition

Major incidents can be:
- Simple or compound
- Compensated or uncompensated
- Natural or man made

Most incidents are:
  Simple (environment intact)
  Compensated (patient load less than capacity available)
  Man made

Equipment

Protective clothing should meet British standards and the current recommendations of the Ambulance Policy Advisory Group. For example, the helmet should be Kevlar composite, green with white lettering, with a visor and chin strap; jackets must be high visibility (motorway standard) and should be clearly labelled in green "DOCTOR" or "NURSE." National standardisation will help recognition at the scene and facilitate control.

Medical supplies are best carried in rucksacks with partitions clearly dividing them into "airway," "breathing," and "circulation." Other rucksacks or boxes that contain only disposable items (airways, dressings, cannulas, and fluids) can be used for resupply. A checklist on the wall of the major incident room will remind team members not to forget important analgesic or anaesthetic drugs from the controlled drugs cupboard or the refrigerator. Specialist operations such as amputations are rarely required and the necessary equipment will not be part of the standard response bag. Consequently it should be stored in a separate mobile surgical team bag together with the equipment needed by the assisting nurse, and kept at the base hospital until needed.

The initial response

A hospital is usually alerted to a major incident by ambulance control, who may either contact the switchboard or speak directly to the accident and emergency department. Standard phrases are used to avoid confusion. *"Major incident, stand by"* is used to warn of a potential incident—perhaps an aircraft about to land with engine trouble. Generally only the senior staff such as the duty consultants in accident and emergency, general surgery, and intensive care need to be told, together with the senior accident and emergency nurse, the duty manager, and the duty nurse administrator. It is wise if these people assemble and establish a *control centre*. Depending on the perceived threat, members of the mobile medical teams can be nominated, change into protective clothing, and check their equipment. When a major incident has been confirmed a full hospital response is initiated by the phrase *"Major incident declared, activate plan."* The response can be terminated at any time by *"Major incident cancelled"* or *"Stand down."*

There will not always be adequate warning from the ambulance service, and it may be the accident and emergency department that activates the plan. In these circumstances ambulance control should be informed.

When a "major incident declared" message is received the following should be established:

- When the accident occurred (time)
- Where it is (including grid reference if known)
- What sort of accident (derailment, aircraft crash, chemical)
- What are the estimated number and severity of casualties
- What medical response is required.

The ambulance incident officer should request a doctor to go to the scene as medical incident officer, together with one or more mobile medical teams. It is not advisable to draw these teams from the hospitals nominated to receive the first casualties. The major incident plan will specify whether the medical incident officer is supplied by a hospital or by a local BASICS (British Association for Immediate Care) scheme. This group of doctors works voluntarily with the emergency services, particularly at road traffic accidents where people are trapped, and their experience may assist with the smooth running of the scene.

Personal protective clothing

- Warm underclothing
- Fire-retardant suit
- High visibility jacket marked "DOCTOR" or "NURSE"
- Hard hat with visor
- Gloves (robust and latex pairs)
- Ear defenders

Additional essential equipment
Everybody
 Personal identification and money
 Notebook (ideally plasticised with water-resistant pen)
 Action card
Medical Incident Officer
 Radio and spare battery
 (Optional:
  Aide memoire
  Camera
  Dictaphone
  Cellular telephone)

Initial information to be passed from the scene

Exact location
Type of incident (road? rail? aircraft?)
Hazards (present and potential)
Access to the scene
Number and severity of casualties (estimate)
Emergency services present and required

Site organisation

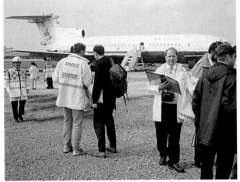

Training for medical command.

Command and control

The overall control of the scene is the responsibility of the police, who will place a secure cordon around it. A second, inner cordon may also be established round the immediate incident if it is necessary to control people moving into a hazardous area. Each emergency service will appoint a commander or incident officer, usually a senior officer. Incident officers will be found near their emergency control vehicles, which should be the only vehicles at the scene that do not switch off their coloured beacons. The incident officers can be regarded as forming "silver command" and their chief officers (who will meet remote from the scene) as "gold command." Forward incident officers will be appointed to control the rescue work at the heart of the incident. If the incident is spread over a large area it will be broken into sectors, each of which will have its own set of forward incident officers referred to as "bronze commanders."

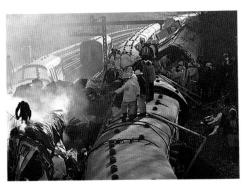

Clapham rail disaster.

The police

As well as securing the scene the police will clear routes in and out of the incident, control the public and volunteers, liaise with the media, activate the voluntary societies (such as the Women's Royal Voluntary Service, the Salvation Army, the St John's Ambulance Service, and the Red Cross), set up a casualty bureau to collate information about the casualties and the dead, identify the dead and organise their removal from the scene, and protect the forensic evidence.

The fire service

If there is a fire or chemical hazard the senior fire officer will assume control of the immediate scene and is responsible for the rescue of any casualties. The fire service also provides specialist equipment and skills to release trapped casualties, as well as emergency lighting and heavy lifting gear.

The ambulance service

The ambulance incident officer will liaise closely with the medical incident officer throughout. It is important that those with specialist paramedical skills are identified and given appropriate tasks. There are a number of key roles for ambulance personnel including a loading officer (to record the destination of casualties), a primary triage officer (to sort the casualties into priorities when they are first found), a casualty clearing station officer (to set up the clearing station), a safety officer (to identify hazards and check personal protective equipment), and a communications officer. It is the ambulance incident officer's duty to nominate the receiving hospitals and arrange provision of the medical incident officer and the mobile medical teams.

The medical service

The medical incident officer is responsible for all medical resources at the scene. Discipline is essential and all members of the mobile medical teams or individual doctors (no matter how senior) will take their instructions from him. As doctors arrive they will be appointed to key roles including triage officer (who may initially be sent forward, then withdrawn to the clearing station), casualty clearing station officer in charge, treatment officers (based at the clearing station), forward medical incident officer, and mortuary officer.

When more than one mobile medical team with nurses is present, a nursing incident officer may be appointed who is responsible to the medical incident officer and who oversees the welfare of the nurses. Members of each mobile medical team must report to the medical incident officer on arrival to be given their jobs. It is usual to concentrate those doctors and nurses used for treatment at the clearing station and send them forward only for specific tasks; otherwise command and control is lost.

> **Standard major incident phrases**
>
> Major incident – standby
> *A major incident is imminent. Warn key staff, and assemble the Hospital Coordination Team*
>
> Major incident declared – activate plan
> *The incident has occurred. A full response is required*
>
> Major incident – cancelled
> *There is no longer the threat of a major incident*
>
> Major incident – stand down
> *The response to an actual incident can now be terminated*

Responsibilities of the medical incident officer

> **Responsibilities of the Medical Incident Officer**
>
> **C**ommand
> **S**afety
> **C**ommunications
> **A**ssessment
> **T**riage
> **T**reatment
> **T**ransport
>
> "Control Spells Calm And Time To Treat"

The medical incident officer has seven principal areas of responsibility.

1 Command and control

This is the cornerstone of efficient management. It can be greatly simplified by reference to the *Prehospital Emergency Management Master*, a waterproof scene guide which doubles as the incident log.[2] A log is essential to compile the report after the incident.

2 Safety

Always consider your own safety first—are you correctly dressed? Next think of the safety of the scene—is it safe to approach and is my team safe? The medical incident officer is responsible for preventing access of any doctor or nurse inappropriately dressed (if they have not been spotted already by the ambulance safety officer). Finally, think of the safety of the casualties.

Major incidents

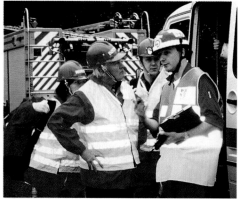

Medical incident officer briefing mobile medical team.

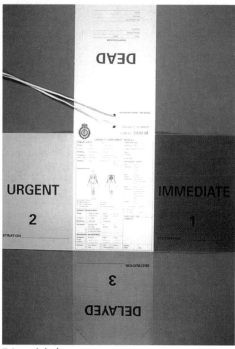

Triage label.

3 Communications

This is the weakest link in the major incident response. All the incident officers must liaise regularly, but the ambulance and medical incident officers should be almost inseparable. The medical incident officer must also relay information to the receiving hospitals. The radio is the usual tool of communication and a knowledge of radio voice procedure will be assumed. At the least you must know how to start and finish a message and how to spell using the phonetic alphabet. Do not forget the value of a runner, particularly when the radio is busy and difficult to get to. Use written messages to avoid "Chinese whispers:" "I need Entonox" could become "I need an empty box."

4 Assessment

This is the assessment of the scene for hazards to your team, and an estimation of the number and severity of casualties. This permits an appropriate early medical response.

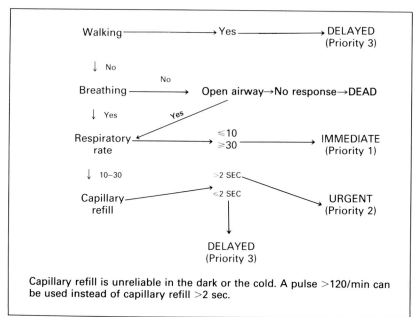

Triage sieve.

5 Triage

Triage is the sorting of casualties into priorities for treatment and specifically those who require immediate treatment (for example, tension pneumothorax), urgent treatment (for example, fractured femur), those whose treatment can be delayed (for example, sprained ankle), and the dead. These priorities are colour coded red, yellow, green, and white, respectively. The triage officer must not stop to treat individual patients. As priorities can change after or while awaiting treatment, triage must be constantly repeated. Colour coded folding labels permit this to be done quickly. The task will be delegated, but supervised, by the medical incident officer.

When dealing with a lot of casualties the aim is to do the most for the most. Consequently there will be a small number who are identified as likely to die. These patients will distract resources from those who are likely to live, and are given minimal treatment initially. They are termed "expectant." Their colour code is green (some use blue), but with the card endorsed "expectant."

Triage can be thought of as an initial rapid assessment, perhaps taking only 30 seconds,

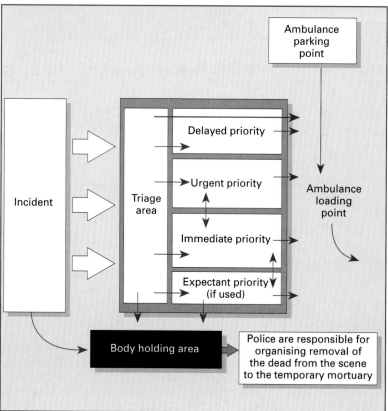

known as the triage sieve. This is followed by a more detailed assessment (usually done at the clearing station) known as the triage sort, for which the triage revised trauma score is used. This gives a score of 0–4 for each of its three components—systolic blood pressure, Glasgow coma scale, and respiratory rate. Triage priorities can be assigned depending on the total score which ranges from 0–12.

6 Treatment

Treatment is always delegated by the medical incident officer and most will take place in the casualty clearing station. The temptation to delay movement of untrapped casualties to the clearing station where the procedures can be done more easily should be avoided. Priorities for treatment follow the rules of airway, breathing, and circulation. Those needing only minor treatment may not receive it at the scene.

7 Transport

The ambulance service is responsible for transporting injured patients to hospital. To decide the most appropriate transport the medical incident officer should consider its capacity, availability, and suitability (such as access to difficult terrain). Before the patient is loaded into the ambulance it should also have been decided which hospital is most appropriate (can the patient go directly to a specialist centre?), what observations and treatment will be required on the way, and if the patient should be escorted.

In addition to these seven areas of responsibility the medical incident officer will monitor the medical response to ensure that it is adequate and that there is a continuing supply of equipment. He will observe team members for signs of fatigue, and organise relief staff usually every four hours. A debrief of all medical personnel involved at the scene should be held within 24 hours.

Patient transport

When choosing the transport think of:

Capacity (a bus may be suitable for large numbers of "delayed" priority casualties)

Availability (save the emergency ambulances for the seriously injured)

Suitability (do you need a wheeled or a tracked vehicle? Is a helicopter more suitable?)

When you have loaded a patient:

Move to the appropriate hospital (are you going straight to a specialist centre?)

Observe in transit (what equipment do you need?)

Verify the treatment before departure (do you have enough oxygen, fluids, or analgesia?)

Escort if necessary (doctor, nurse, or paramedic?)

Hospital organisation

The key to successful hospital management of a major incident is, once again, command and control. It depends on the early establishment of an effective control centre staffed by senior hospital medical, nursing, and administrative coordinators with appropriate support staff. All should be of the most senior rank possible (for example, a consultant, a senior nursing officer, and a senior administrator) and be thoroughly familiar with the major incident plan.

Other personnel should also be aware of their roles in the response to a major incident, but to anticipate a lack of familiarity (and to assist junior staff) everybody should be issued with an "action card" when they report for duty. These will be distributed according to clinical need rather than personal choice.

Actions on receiving "Major incident – standby"

Medical, nursing and administrative coordinators meet and establish the control centre. They then:

- Liaise with the ambulance service about the details and status of the incident
- Nominate the medical incident officer and dispatch him or her to the scene, if appropriate
- Start to prepare the accident and emergency department for the reception of casualties
- Warn theatres, the intensive care unit, and outpatients about the possible disruption of activities
- Establish an accurate bed state

Actions on receiving "Major incident declared – activate plan"

Coordinators meet and establish the control centre, if no prior warning. They then:

- Dispatch the medical incident officer to the scene
- Establish whether mobile medical teams are required; collect the teams, ensure the members are properly clothed and equipped, and dispatch them to the scene
- Establish a triage point
- Clear the accident and emergency department of existing casualties and prepare for the reception of casualties
- Inform theatres and outpatients that normal activities must be suspended; ask the intensive care unit to clear beds if possible
- Designate a ward for the reception of admitted casualties and start emptying it of existing patients
- Organise staff as they arrive
- Arrange facilities for the police, relatives, and the media

---

Medical coordinator

The immediate priorities of the medical coordinator are to clear the accident and emergency department, to dispatch the medical incident officer if requested from that hospital, and to organise the mobile medical teams, ensuring that they are appropriately dressed and equipped and have transport to the scene. The medical coordinator should check that the switchboard operators are calling in appropriate staff from home and the hospital residences, and he must nominate a senior doctor to be *chief triage officer*. This doctor receives casualties at the ambulance entrance and reassesses their treatment priority before allocating them to a treatment area within the department.

The clinical activity is supervised by the *surgical triage officer* (usually the duty consultant surgeon) and where needed the *medical triage officer* (the duty consultant physician or intensive care specialist). Surgical triage must take account of not only which patient has priority, but what operation has priority for each patient; those that are life saving should be done first.

The medical coordinator (or a deputy, the team coordinator) will form doctors and nurses into either treatment or transfer teams, and allocate them to appropriate areas of the department. Many of the staff in the accident and emergency department will be drawn from other areas in the hospital. It is important that regular accident and emergency staff can be identified by tabards to help the unfamiliar staff find equipment and supplies.

With the help of the nursing coordinator an accurate bed state, including intensive care beds, must be maintained, together with available operating theatre resources. Staff welfare must be monitored and refreshments ordered. At intervals the medical coordinator may be requested by the administrators to address a press conference.

Nursing coordinator

The nursing coordinator will recruit nurses to go with the mobile medical teams and to attend patients in the accident and emergency department. One nurse should be provided for each stretcher patient although up to four may be required for the resuscitation of a critically ill patient if resources allow. The nursing coordinator should liaise closely with the medical coordinator.

Administrative coordinator

To run a hospital's major incident response successfully requires a great deal of documentation and record keeping, firstly to keep track of patients (particularly if they are to be discharged); secondly to provide the police with information for their documentation team (one of whom is sent to each receiving hospital to report to the central casualty bureau); and thirdly to answer questions from relatives who arrive at the hospital. The administrative coordinator must: allocate a room for the police documentation team, ideally with a telephone and facsimile machine; and organise a media centre remote from the accident and emergency department where the press can be briefed at regular intervals.

Porters and security staff must be organised to ensure that patients are transported expeditiously and that unwanted people are kept out of the treatment areas. Space for relatives must be set aside, together with a room in which to talk to the bereaved.

The aftermath

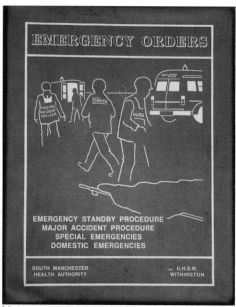

Major incident plan.

When the medical or ambulance incident officer reports that the last casualty has left the site, and when all patients have been either admitted to or discharged from the accident and emergency department the medical coordinator will declare a "stand down" of the major incident procedure.

Debriefing is essential. An "emotional" debriefing should be organised within 24 hours so that all the departmental staff have a chance to express their feelings. If proper opportunities are not given to staff for debriefing and counselling some are likely to develop symptoms of post-traumatic stress disorder. Heads of departments should prepare formal reports which can be used to improve the Major Incident Plan.

1 NHS Management Executive. *Emergency planning in the NHS: Health Services arrangements for dealing with major incidents.* London: HMSO, 1990.
2 Hodgetts TJ, McNeil I, Cooke MW. *The prehospital emergency management master.* London: BMJ Publishing Group, 1995.

Further reading
Hodgetts TJ, Mackway-Jones K. *Major incident medical management and support: the practical approach.* London: BMJ Publishing Group, 1995.

The photograph of the Clapham disaster by Frank Spooner Pictures.

INDEX

abbreviated injury scale 83
ABCDE approach 2–5
abdomen
    radiography 51
    reflex 45
    rigidity 50
abdominal trauma
    assessment 8, 43, 49–50
    blunt 49, 53, 54
    children 104–5
    elderly 110
    information required 50
    investigations 51
    laparotomy 51
    management 53
    pelvic injuries 63
    penetrating 49, 53, 95
    peritoneal lavage 52
    tetraplegia 43
accident scene 60, 115
    analgesia 114
    chemical incidents 125
    clothing 111
    entrapment 113
    indications for transportation 112
    major incidents 136–7
    nurses 81
    observation 111
    primary survey 112–13
    records 114
    safety 111
acetabular fracture 61, 78
acid–base analysis 17
acidosis 16, 17, 22, 66, 93
Addisonian crisis 68
administrative coordinator 140
air emboli 127
airway 2–3, 16, 17, 42, 112, 115, 132
    anaesthesia 13
    burn patients 118–19, 120
    children 98–9
    elderly 107
    first vital minutes 11
    hospital management 12
    intubation technique 13–14
    maxillofacial injuries 36–7
    nurse 80
    oxygenation and ventilation 12
    pregnancy 93
    premorbid conditions 66
airway injury 21
airway obstruction 3, 6, 11, 29, 36–7
airway resistance 20
albumin (HPPF) 101
alcohol 13, 35, 70
allergies 70
alternating current 123
altitude 134
Ambulance Policy Advisory Group 135
ambulance service 1, 136, 137
ambulances 116–17
amnesia 32

ampicillin 68
AMPLE history 70, 110
amputation, traumatic 64, 128
amylase, serum 51
anaemia 68–9
anaesthetics 13, 31, 114
anal reflex 45
analgesics 10, 26, 33, 35, 43, 106, 114, 119
anatomical scoring system 83
angiography 79
ankle fractures 61, 63
ankylosing spondylitis 66
antibiotics 48, 56, 62, 68, 130
    head injury 31, 33, 34
anxiety 35
aortic injuries 7, 19, 20, 77, 104
aortic valve disease 68
aortocaval compression syndrome 93
apnoea 3, 11, 12
arm
    areflexia 45
    fractures 63
Armback splint 116
arterial lines 17, 101
arteriography 61
    renal 55
assessment see initial assessment; radiological
    assessment
asthma 67
atelectasis 18, 20
atlanto-odontoid gap 46
atlas
    fracture 46, 74
    transverse ligament rupture 46
atracurium 13, 31
atropine 42, 43
autonomic dysfunction 69
axonal injury 28

back wounds 53
bad news, breaking 88, 89–90
    staff reaction 92
bag–valve face mask 11
barbiturates 11
Beck's triad 19
Beevor's sign 44
benzylpenicillum 33
bereavement care (CRUSE) 92
beta₂ agonists 119
beta blockers 23, 43
biochemical tests 34, 51
bladder injuries 57, 78
blast
    injuries 127–8, 129–30
    lung 128
    waves 127–8
    winds 128
blood
    autologous 25
    count 4, 33, 51
    crossmatching 4, 17, 51, 101
    filters 25

gas tensions 4, 12, 14, 17, 19, 26, 33, 43,
    50, 66, 119
glucose 34
blood loss 4
    classification of hypovolaemic shock 22
    control 4, 23
    effects 22
    fractures 60
    occult 67
    pregnancy 93
    replacement 23–5
    response 22–3
blood pressure 4, 9, 16, 29, 33
    blood loss 22–3
    children 23, 100
blood transfusion 17, 25, 119
blood volume 4, 108
    children 100
    pregnancy 93
blunt trauma 1
    abdomen 49, 53, 54
    neck 37
    pregnancy 95
body temperature 70, 102
bomb injuries
    management 129–30
    mechanisms 127–8
    penetrating missiles 129
bombs, unexploded 126
bone
    facial 38
    loose fragments 38, 65
    radiology 73, 76, 78
bowel
    blast injury 128
    exposed 8, 53
    sounds 50
brachial plexus injury 45
brachial vein 24
bradycardia 13, 29
    shock 43
brain damage 102
    diffuse 28
    focal impact 29
    haematomas 29
    hypoxia and ischaemia 29
    raised intracranial pressure 29
brain shifts 30
brainstem compression 30
breathing 3–4, 16, 112, 132
    children 99
    diaphragmatic 44
    elderly 108
    laboured 21
    pregnancy 93
    premorbid conditions 66–7
British Association of Immediate
    Care 115, 136
bronchial injuries 21, 77, 104
bronchial intubation 14
bronchitis 67
bronchoscopy 21, 37

Index

bronchospasm 67
Brown–Séquard syndrome 44
bulbar injuries 57
bulbocavernosus reflex 45
bullet wounds 49, 129, 130
burns 67
  airway 118, 120
  analgesia and reassurance 120
  assessment 119, 121
  chemical 122
  children 106
  dressing 121
  drug contraindications 13
  electrical 120, 123
  escharotomy 121
  flash 123, 128
  fluid requirements 119, 121
  intravenous access 119
  lethal 121
  pregnancy 95
  preparation for transfer to hospital 118
  reassessment 120–2
  reception and resuscitation 118
  transfer 122
  urine 120
burr holes 34

calcium 17
  gluconate 122
Canada 125
cannulation, arterial 17, 101
cannulation, intravenous 4, 23–4, 119
  cervical injury 43
  children 101
capillary return 61
capnography 14
carbolic acid 122
carbon monoxide poisoning 120
carboxyhaemoglobin concentrations 119, 122
  calculation 120
cardiac arrest 42, 43, 116
cardiac arrhythmias 7, 68, 104, 108, 122, 123
cardiac contractility 26
cardiac contusions 7, 20, 104
cardiac failure 26
cardiac injuries 17, 19, 77
cardiac output 16
  elderly 108
  pregnancy 93
cardiac pacemakers 68
cardiac rupture 20
cardiac tamponade 3, 16, 17, 26, 104
  management 18–19
cardiac transplants 69
cardiac valves
  avulsion 20
  disease 68
  donation 91
cardiotocography 94, 95
cardiovascular response
  drugs modifying 70
  elderly 108
carotid arteries 21, 38
cartilage (radiology) 73, 76, 78
catecholamines 22, 23, 26
catherisation, urethral 43, 51, 57, 58
cefuroxime 62
central nervous system 5, 69, 102, 108, 113
central venous pressure 4, 17, 25, 26, 43, 120
  access 24
  children 101
  elderly 108
cephadrine 56
cephalic vein 24
cerebral function 12
cerebral hypoxia 22
cerebral ischaemia 29, 102
cerebral oedema 69, 102
cerebral perfusion pressure 30
cerebrospinal fluid 6, 30, 39
cerebrovascular disease 69
cervical fascia 19

cervical spine
  children 103
  important measurements 73
  protection 2–3, 11, 41, 42, 98, 107, 112, 113, 132
cervical spine injuries 12, 41, 42, 44, 47
  classification 73
  cord damage 41, 42, 43, 44, 72, 73
  hyperextension/hyperflexion 74
  instability 72, 73
  neurological damage 72, 74
  premorbid medical problems 66–7, 73
  radiological assessment 7, 45–6, 72–5
cervical spondylosis 44, 46
cervicothoracic junction 45, 73
cheek swelling 38
chemical burns 122
chemical hazards 124
chemical incidents 124–6
  delayed symptoms 125
chest
  examination 3, 7
  flail 3, 18, 76, 104
  pain 18, 20
  radiographs 14, 17, 19, 33, 37, 51
chest drain 4, 11, 67, 116
  insertion 17
chest injuries 53, 110
  children 104
  deaths 15
  life threatening 15–19
  pathophysiology 16
  potentially lethal 20–21
  primary survey 3, 16
  radiological assessment 75–7
  resuscitation 17
  secondary survey 7, 19
  type 15
chest wall
  examination 7
  injuries 15, 18, 76, 104
childhood trauma
  airway 98–9
  breathing 99
  burns 106
  causes 97
  circulation and control of bleeding 100–1
  dysfunction and exposure 102
  equipment 98
  head 102–3
  non-accidental injury 106
  pain relief 23, 106
  renal 54, 105
  resuscitation chart 97
  secondary survey 102–5
  skeletal and soft tissue injuries 105
children 23, 90
  anatomical differences 98
  vital signs: normal values 101
chin lift 11
chloramphenicol 34, 39
chlordiazepoxide 70
circulation 4, 16, 113, 133
  children 100
  elderly 108
  nurse 81
  pregnancy 93
  premorbid conditions 67–9
  spinal cord trauma 43
clonazepam 33
clostridial infection 130
clothing, protective 1, 111, 135
coagulation problems 25
coagulopathy 69
cocaine 13
Cocodamol 33
colloid solutions 4, 24–5, 119, 133
coma 34, 69, 109
  chart 30, 45
  deaths 35
  intracranial pressure 30
  position 41
  scale 84, 102

compartment syndromes 64
Compassionate Friends 92
computed tomography 32, 51, 55, 63, 77, 79, 103, 105, 109
concussion 28
  postconcussion symptoms 35
confusion 22, 109, 110, 115
"coning" 30
conscious level
  assessment 5, 6, 30
  deterioration 33–4
copper sulphate 122
corneal reflex 6
corneas 91
coronary artery disease 23
cortisol, serum 68
cost–benefit analysis 83
cotrimoxazole 31, 33
cranial nerves 35, 39
cribriform plate injury 11, 39
cricoid 12, 14, 98
cricothyroidotomy 11, 12, 99, 132
CRUSE (bereavement care) 92
crush injuries 128
crystalloid solutions 24, 119, 133
Curling's ulcers 67
Cushing's ulcers 67
cyanide poisoning 120
cyanosis 11, 16
Cyclimorph 120
cystogram 8, 57

dantrolene 69
deaf patients 110
deaths from injury 15, 53, 63, 66, 104
  probability 85
debriefing 81–2, 92, 139, 140
decontamination 125
decubitus ulcers 109
dehydration 34, 69
dentures 107
depression after minor head injury 35
desert 134
DF118 33
diabetes mellitus 69
diaphragmatic injury 7, 19, 21, 76, 104
diazepam 26, 33, 103
dicobalt edetate 120
dihydrocodeine 33
Diploma in Immediate Medical Care 135
diplopia 39
disability (definition) 87
disasters 134
disc spaces 73
dislocations 61, 62, 74, 76
disseminated intravascular coagulation 95
diuretics 67, 69
dizziness 35
dobutamine 26
documentation 10, 114, 117
  nurse 81
dopamine 26
drugs contraindicated in trauma 13
dysfunction (CNS) 5, 69, 102, 108, 113

eardrum rupture 127
ears, bleeding from 39
elbow fractures 105
elderly
  AMPLE history 110
  blood loss 23
  cardiovascular changes 108
  lung function 108
  primary survey and resuscitation 107–9
  renal function 108
  secondary survey 109–110
electrical burns 120, 123
electrocardiography 4, 7, 16, 19, 33, 68, 103, 104, 122
electrolytes 34, 51, 68
  premorbid imbalance 69
embolisation 79
Emergency Planning in the NHS 135

empathy 90
emphysema 67
  surgical 19, 21, 37, 39, 76, 77
endoscopy 12
endotracheal intubation *see* intubation
energy transfer 109, 115, 129
enophthalmos 39
Entonox 10, 26, 114, 120
entrapment 113–14
environment 70
  hostile 131–4
epiglottis 98
  swelling 118
epilepsy 29
escharotomy 121
ethanol 13
ethmoids 38
ethylene glycol 122
etomidate 31
exophthalmos 39
explosions 127–8
exposure 5, 113
  children 102
  elderly 109
extraction devices 113
extradural haematoma 29, 102
extremities 8
  see also limb injuries
eye movements 39
eyes
  chemical irritation 125
  examination 6, 39
  injuries 13, 39

face
  cleaning 38
  examination 6, 39
  palpation 40
  trauma 12, 38, 39, 40
facial artery 38
falls
  children 97
  from height 54, 55, 61
fat emboli 67
femoral fractures 61, 63
femoral vein 24
fetomaternal haemorrhage 94
fetus 93
  assessment 94
  distress 94
  injury 95
fire service 113, 118, 124, 137
fits 69
flail chest 3, 18, 76, 104
flank 53, 55
flash burns 123, 128
fluid replacement 4, 17, 23–5, 43, 113
  burns 119–20, 121
  children 101
  coagulation problems 25
  elderly 108
  hostile environments 133
  valvular disease 68
Foote Hospital, Florida 81
Foundation for the Study of Infant Deaths 92
fractures
  blood loss 60
  closed 64
  compression 61
  elderly 109, 110
  epiphyseal 105
  management 63, 64–5
  open 64–5
  radiology 71–2
  see also specific fractures
fragmentation missiles 128
frontozygomatic suture 39
fundoscopy 39, 45

gag reflex 11, 98
Gardner–Wells caliper 47
gases, toxic 120

gastric contents
  aspiration 12, 104
  leaking 21
gastric distension 8
gastric intubation 11, 42, 51
  children 99
gelofusine 25
genitalia 59
gentamicin 62, 68
Glasgow coma scale 30, 84
  children 102
gloves, protective 1
grief reactions 89, 92
Guedel airway 3, 42
gum elastic bougie 12, 14
gunshot wounds 53, 54, 56, 129, 130

Haemaccel 25, 94
haematomas, 21, 72, 78
  see also specific haematomas
haematuria 55
haemoglobin 50, 63, 99
haemoglobinopathies 68–9
haemoglobinuria 120
haemopericardium 77
haemopneumothorax 19
haemoptysis 21, 104
haemorrhage
  children 100
  control 4, 23, 37, 38, 60, 108, 113, 133
  intra-abdominal 8
  on removal of tamponade 17, 19
haemothorax 4, 18
halothane 13
handicap (definition) 87
Hangman's fracture 75
Hartmann's solution 4
headache 35
head injuries 6, 17, 133
  aims of management 29
  brain damage 28–30
  characteristics of patients 28
  children 102–3
  conscious level deterioration 33–4
  drugs 13, 33
  elderly 109
  hospital admission 32–3
  incidence 29
  interhospital transfer 34
  intubation 12, 31
  management 30–2
  minor 35
  outcome 35
  warning card 32
Health Service Guidelines 124
heart *see* cardiac
heart rate, child 101
Heimlich valves 132
helicopter transport 116–17
hepatitis viruses 1
Hetastarch 25
high energy transfer injuries 129, 130
hippocampal neurones 29
HIV 1
hostile environment
  evacuation 134
  guidelines 131–2
  head injuries 133
  particular problems 134
  resuscitation 132–3
hydrocortisone 67, 68
hydrofluoric acid 122
hydrogen
  chloride 120
  cyanide 120
  sulphide 120
hypercapnia 12
hyperkalaemia 69
hypernatraemia 69
hyperpyrexia, malignant 69
hypertension 68
  renal 56
hypocalcaemia 69

hypoglycaemia 69, 70
hyponatraemia 69
hypotension 9, 13, 22, 23
  brain damage 29, 33
  ischaemic heart disease 68
  neurogenic 43, 44
  premorbid 67–8
hypothermia 69, 70, 109, 113, 118
hypovolaemic shock 13, 60, 116
  cardiac contractility and urine output 26
  children 100
  classification 22
  haemorrhage control 23
  monitoring 25–6
  pain relief 26
  pathophysiology 22
  pneumatic counter pressure suit 27, 116
  pregnancy 93–5
  pulmonary oxygenation 23
  replacement of blood loss 23–5
  symptoms and signs 4, 22–3
hypoxaemia 11, 12
hypoxia 11, 12, 14, 17, 22, 43, 67
  brain damage 29, 33
  indications 16

ileus 42, 43, 55
impairment (definition) 87
initial assessment 81
  prehospital information 2
  primary survey and resuscitation 2–5
  reassessment 10
  reception and transfer 2
  secondary survey 6–9
  trauma team 1–2
Injury Impairment Scale 86
injury severity score 83
inotropic drugs 26, 43
intercanthal distance 39
intercostal drainage 17
interhospital transfer 117
  head injuries 34
intracranial haematoma 28, 29, 32, 34
intracranial infection 29, 33
intracranial pressure 39
  drugs increasing 13
  laryngoscopy 13
  mannitol 33
  raised 29, 30, 68, 101, 103, 133
intradural haematoma 29
intraosseous infusion 100
intraperitoneal injury 50
intravenous cannulation *see* cannulation
intravenous fluids *see* fluid replacement
intubation 3, 11, 12, 37, 42, 66, 112, 118
  children 99
  equipment 13
  head injuries 31
  technique 13–14
ischaemia
  cerebral 29
  distal 61
ischaemic heart disease 67, 68, 108, 122

jaw angle 98
jaw thrust 11
Jefferson fracture (atlas) 46, 74
joints 61
  radiology 72, 73, 76, 78
jugular vein 21, 38
  cannulation 24, 101
jungle 134

Kendrick Extraction Device 113
ketamine 13, 26, 114
kinetic energy 129
Kleihaur test 94
Kussmaul's sign 19

lacrimal apparatus 39
laparotomy 51, 53, 63
laryngeal reflex 11
laryngoscopy 13–14

Index

children 99
complication 13
larynx 37
children 98
injuries 21, 37
last meal 70
life expectancy 107
lightning 123
limb injuries 23
assessment 8, 61
compartment syndromes 64
fracture management 64–5
haemorrhage 60
neurological state 62
pelvis 62–3
prehospital care 60
radiology 63
splintage 63, 116
traumatic amputation 64
vascular state 61
wound management 62
liver, ruptured 25, 53
log rolling 9
loins 55
low energy transfer injuries 129, 130
lumbar puncture 34
lumbar vertebrae 51, 55
Lund and Browder chart 121
lung, blast 128
lung compliance 20, 108
lung see also pulmonary

magnetic resonance imaging 48
major incidents
aftermath 140
communication 138
hospital organisation 139–40
initial information 136
medical incident officer 135, 137–9
plan 136, 140
preparation 135–6
site organisation 136–7
staff training 135
standard phrases 137
Major Trauma Outcome Study 86
mandible
fractures 6, 36, 40
palpation 39
mannitol 33, 48
marijuana 13
maxilla
closed injury 38
fractures 36, 39, 40
maxillofacial injuries
airway management 36–7
management of bleeding 38
secondary survey 38–40
maxillofacial radiographs 40
mediastinum 19, 37, 47
air 19, 76, 77
injuries 77
mobility in children 104
medical antishock trousers 4, 27, 94, 104, 116
medical coordinator (major incident) 139–40
medical history 9, 70
medical incident officer
responsibilities 137–9
training 135
medical problems (premorbid) 122
AMPLE history 70
assessment and management 66–9
prevalence and effect 66
meningitis 6, 34, 39
mesenteric injury 49
metacarpal fractures 8
metatarsal fractures 8
methylprednisolone 48
metoclopramide 26, 33
midazolam 26
missile injuries 21, 54, 128, 129–30
morphine 10, 26, 106, 114
mortality see deaths from injury
motor cyclists 41, 45

mouth-to-face mask 11
muscle relaxants 13, 31, 114
mydriasis 39
myocardium
contusion 7, 20, 104
impaired 26
infarction 68, 122
myoglobinuria 120

nalbuphine 13, 26
narcotics 43
nasal prongs 98
nasal septum 38
nasal see also nose
nasoethmoidal fracture 39
nasogastric intubation 11, 42, 51
nasopharyngeal airway 3, 132
nasotracheal intubation 12, 13
National Poisons Unit 124, 125, 126
nausea 33
neck
blunt trauma 37
burns 121
children 103, 104
collars 41, 42, 113
examination 3, 7, 37
immobilisation 41
radiographs 37
stiffness 34
veins 16, 18, 67
wounds 38
nephrectomy 56
nerve blocks 114
neurogenic shock 9, 43
neuroleptic malignant syndrome 69
neurological diseases 69
neurological examination 6, 9, 43–4, 62, 133
unconscious patient 45
neurological recovery 35
neuropathies 109
neurosurgical consultation 32
non-accidental injury 106
North Western Injury Research Centre 87
nose
bleeding 37, 38
examination 39
packing 38
nurses 80–2, 137
nursing coordinator 140

odontoid fracture 46, 75
oedema 23, 37
oesophageal injuries 7, 21, 77
open fractures 64–5
opiate agonists 13
opiates 13, 26, 33, 114
opioids 120
oral cavity
bleeding 38
cleaning 38
haematoma 40
orbit 39
organ donation 91
oropharyngeal suction 42
oropharynx 37
orotracheal intubation 3, 12, 37, 66
children 99
outcome 86
oxygen
administration 3, 11, 67, 108, 112, 116, 119, 132
children 98, 99
delivery 17
hyperbaric 120
saturation 25
tension 108
oxygenation 12, 23, 43

pacemakers 68
packed cell volume 25, 51, 101
paediatric trauma see childhood trauma
pain relief 10, 26, 114
burns 120

children 23, 106
head injuries 33
pancreatic injury 51
pancuronium 13
paracetamol 33
paralysis, flaccid 44
paraplegia 43, 48
paravertebral haematoma 47, 50
parotid duct 39
pelvis
assessment 8, 50
fractures 50, 57, 58, 62, 78, 94, 105
injuries 62–3
radiological assessment 77–8
stabilisation 62
pelviureteric junction
disruption 54
treatment 56
penetrating wounds 18, 49, 50, 53, 54, 95, 128, 129–30
penicillin 31, 34
penile injury 59
peptic ulcer disease 67
pericardial effusion 68
see also cardiac tamponade
pericardiocentesis 19, 26, 68
perinephric haematoma 55
perineum 8
peripheral nerves
division 62
ischaemia 61
peritoneal lavage 8, 43, 53, 63, 94, 105
procedure 52
peritoneum 50, 53
phaeochromocytoma 68
phalangeal fractures 8
pharynx
palpation of wall 38
reflex 11
stimulation 42
phenol 122
phenoxymethylpenicillin 33
phenytoin 33, 103
photography
accident scene 111
wound 62
physiological scoring systems 84
placental abruption 93, 95
platysma 7
pleural effusions 67, 76
pneumatic counter pressure suit 4, 27, 94, 104, 116
pneumomediastinum 19, 76, 77
pneumothorax
open 11, 18
tension 4, 11, 17, 21, 26, 76, 104, 108, 112, 114, 116
poisons centres 124
telephone numbers 126
polygelatins 24–5
Portex Emergency drainage bags 132
post-traumatic stress disorder 92, 128, 140
predental space 73
pregnancy
anatomical changes 93
blunt and penetrating trauma 95
burns 95
hospital admission 95
physiological changes 93
Rh negative mothers 94
surveys 94
prehospital care
accident scene 60, 111–14, 115
limb injuries 60
transportation 115–17, 139
Prehospital Emergency Care Certificate 135
Prehospital Emergency Management Master 137
premorbid medical conditions 66–70
pressure sores 109
prevertebral haematoma 46
priapism 8, 44
primary survey 2–5
airway management 2

breathing   3
circulation and haemorrhage control   4
dysfunction of central nervous system   5
exposure   5
propanolol   20
propofol   31
proptosis   39
prostate gland   50, 58
protective clothing   1, 111, 135
psychometric testing   35
psychotherapy   35
pubic ramus fracture   50, 77, 78
pubic symphysis   57, 58
disruption   50, 58, 77, 78
pulmonary arteries   20
pulmonary artery wedge pressure   26
pulmonary collapse   76
pulmonary contusions   7, 20, 76, 104
pulmonary emboli   67
pulmonary laceration   19
pulmonary oedema   43, 67, 76
pulmonary ventilation   3–4, 23
pulse   4, 16, 22, 25, 33, 68
distal   61
pulse oximetry   4, 13, 14, 43, 113, 119
pupils   39
pyelography   8, 105

radio communication   138
radiological assessment   10, 71
ABC's system   72
cervical spine   45–6, 72–5
chest   75–7
limbs   63
pelvis   77–9
pregnancy   94
skull   79
thoracolumbar spine   47
reassessment of patient   10
reception of patient   2, 117
recovery position   41
rectal examination   8, 50
relatives and friends   10
action in event of death   91
arrival at hospital   89
bad news   89–90
information and follow up   91–2
initial contact   88
nurse   81
room   89
seeing body after death   91
seeing patient   90–1
support organisations   92
renal arteriography   55
renal artery thrombosis   56
renal failure   69
renal function   120
renal injuries   8, 104
classification   54
clinical presentation   55
late complications   56
management   56
mechanisms   54
radiological investigations   55
silent   56
surgical exploration   56
renal perfusion   4
renal veins   56
respiratory diseases   66–7
respiratory distress syndrome   20, 64
respiratory rate   112
children   100
restlessness   33
resuscitation   2–4, 16, 17, 23, 112–13, 129
children   97–101
elderly   107–9
hypotensive   133
reassessing response   10
room   1, 2
retrobulbar haemorrhage   39
retroperitoneal haematoma   56, 63
retroperitoneal injury   50
retropharyngeal haematoma   44

retropharyngeal space   46
retrotracheal space   46
revised trauma score   84
rheumatoid arthritis   66, 67
rib fractures   7, 8, 11, 18, 19, 47, 51, 55
complications   76
elderly   110
Ringer lactate solution   4, 24
road traffic accidents   49, 50, 61, 97, 136
RoadPeace   92
Russell Extraction Device   113

sacral reflexes   45
safety   111, 129, 137
saline   119
Salter-Harris classification (fractures)   105
Samaritans   92
saphenous vein   24, 119
Savlon   38
scalds   106
scalp   6, 38, 103
scapular fractures   19
scoring systems
anatomical   83
future developments   87
input criteria   83–4
major trauma outcome study   86
objectives   87
output variables   86
physiological   84
TRISS methodology   85
scrotal injuries   59
sea   134
seat belt injuries   49
secondary survey   6–10
objectives   6
sedation   33
seizures   33, 34, 35, 103
Seldinger technique   24
Semtex   127
shock see also hypovolaemic shock
neurogenic   9, 43
septic   67
sickle cell disease   69
skin
assessment   9
colour   61
flaps   65
grafts   65
pallor   22, 23
temperature   61
skull
burr holes   34
radiography   31, 45, 79, 103
traction   47
skull fractures   29, 31, 109
basal   6, 11, 13, 38, 114
children   102, 103
smoke injury   118–19, 128
sodium nitroprusside   20
sodium thiosulphate   120
soft tissue
fragments   38
injuries   9, 38, 65, 105
prevertebral   73
radiography   72, 73, 76, 78
swelling   37
spinal board   42, 113, 115
spinal canal   73
spinal centres   48
spinal cord injuries   13, 41, 42
children   103
circulation   43
complications   43
drug treatment   48
partial lesions   44
radiological evidence   45, 73
signs and symptoms   43, 44
syndromes   44
spinal injuries   5, 61, 94, 132
accident scene   41–2
lifting patient   42
paraplegia and tetraplegia   48

primary survey   42–3
radiology   45–7, 72–5
secondary survey   9, 43–5
treatment   47–8
transfer to hospital   42
spine immobilisers   42, 113
spleen
haematomas   51
rupture   25, 53
splintage   60, 63, 116
stab wounds   49, 53, 54, 55, 56
sternal fractures   18, 20, 47, 76
sternoclavicular joint dislocation   76
steroids   33, 68
spinal cord injury   48
stress   81–2
post-traumatic   92, 128, 140
stroke   69
subclavian arteries   38
subclavian vein, cannulation   24, 43
subconjunctival ecchymosis   39
subdural haematoma   29, 102, 109
submental triangle   98
suction   42
sulphonamides   39
survival probability   85
suxamethonium   13, 31

tachycardia   4, 22, 23, 108
tachypnoea   22
"teardrop fracture"   46, 74
teeth   6, 40
temporal artery   38
temporomandibular joints   66, 107
tension pneumothorax see pneumothorax
testicles   59
tetanus prophylaxis   1, 10, 62, 121, 130
tetraplegia   48
pulse rate   43
respiratory insufficiency   43
thiamine   70
thiopentone   31
thirst   22
thoracic trauma see chest injuries
thoracolumbar spine   47
thoracotomy   16, 21
thrombocytopenia   69
tibial fracture   61, 62, 63
tidal volume in children   99
tissue perfusion   22, 43
TNT   127
tongue
anterior insertion   36
sublingual haematoma   40
tourniquets   4, 23
trachea
deviation   44, 73
injuries   21, 37, 104
length in children   98
tracheobronchial disruption   19
tracheostomy   11, 21, 118
training   81, 135
transportation of patients   139
between hospitals   34, 117
burns   122
communication and handover   117
indications for   111
monitoring   116
packaging and stabilisation   115–16
"Platinum 10 minutes"   115
trauma deaths see deaths from injury
trauma nurses   80–2, 137
trauma sheet   10
trauma team   1, 2, 80–2
triage   138–9
chemical accident   125
hospital   139–40
trimethoprim   56
trinitrotoluene   127
TRISS methodology   85

ultrasonography   51, 55, 63, 79
Doppler   61, 94

Index

umbilicus 44
uncal transtentorial herniation 30
unconscious patients 113
  airway 3, 11, 13, 23, 41
  brain damage 29
  elderly 109
  ischaemic heart disease 68
  neurological examination 45
  spinal examination 44
United States 66
urea 34, 51
ureteric injury 51
ureterogram 55
urethography 58, 63
urethral catheterisation 43, 51, 57, 58
urethral injuries 8, 50, 58
urinary retention 43, 57
urinary tract 63
  lower 57–9
  upper 54–6
urine of burn patients 120
urine output 4, 8, 22, 25, 26, 43, 105, 120
urine testing 8
urography 55, 58
uterus 93
  rupture 95

Vacumat 115
vagal reflex stimulation 42
vaginal examination 50, 94
vascular injuries 17, 77
vascular state 61
vecuronium 13, 31
venous access 4, 24, 133
  burns 119
  children 100

venous cutdown 24, 100, 119, 133
venous pressure, central see central venous
    pressure
ventilation, assisted 3, 11, 12, 67, 116, 132
  children 99
ventricular septal rupture 20
vertebral canal 73
visual acuity 6, 39
vital capacity 43
vomiting 3, 103

white phosphorous 122
wound management 62, 65, 130

zygoma fractures 39
zygomaticomaxillary suture 39

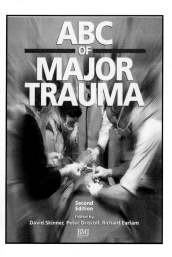
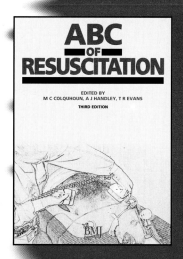
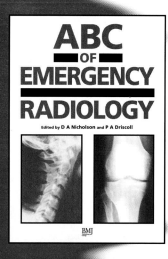
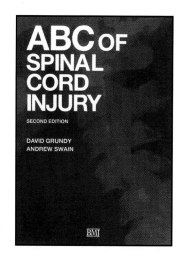
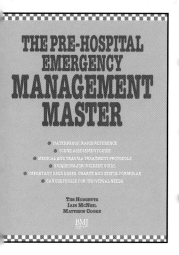
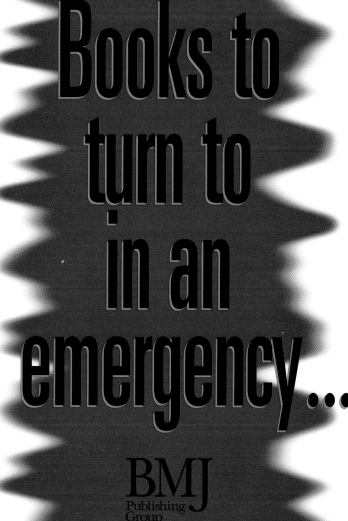
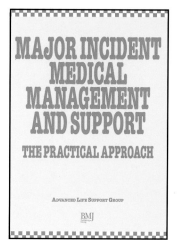
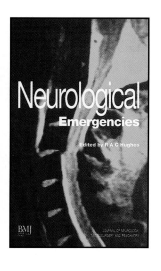
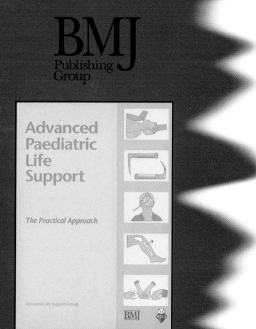
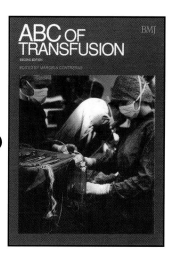
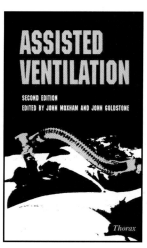
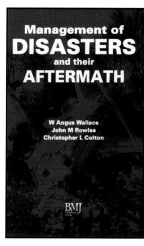